Functional Exercise Progressions

Mary Yoke, MA
Carol Kennedy, MS

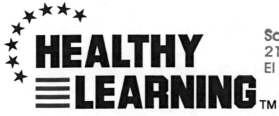

ISBN: 978-1-58518-998-4
Library of Congress Control Number: 2003106969

Book layout: Jennifer Bokelmann
Cover design: Kerry Hartjen
Text and cover photos: Ryan Rudd
Illustrations: Clint Smith. Used by permission of E2 Systems, Inc. — Pages 13, 21, 29, 37, 45, 53, 63, 79 (top and middle), 97 (bottom), 105
Jeanne Hamilton — Pages 71, 79 (bottom), 89, 97 (top), 113

Healthy Learning
P.O. Box 1828
Monterey, CA 93942
www.healthylearning.com

Dedication

To my wonderful sons, Nathaniel and Zachary. —Mary Yoke

To my awesome kids, Tony and Jessica. —Carol Kennedy

Thanks for being patient with us as we took time out of your lives to work on this book. We love you guys!

Acknowledgments

We would like to extend our appreciation to Dr. Larry Golding and Scott Golding for permission to use selected anatomical illustrations from their renowned book, *The Fitness Professionals' Guide to Musculoskeletal Anatomy and Human Movement*. We would also like to thank Indiana University's Division of Recreational Sports for allowing us to use their strength and conditioning equipment for the photo shots. In addition, we would like to thank the following fitness/wellness professional staff who demonstrated the specific exercises in the book: William Thornton, Teri Bladen, Kris Neely, Misty Schneider; Evan McDowell, Chad Coplen, and Cara McGowan.

The following Division of Recreational Sports strength and conditioning consultants and HPER students also assisted us as models in the photo shoot: Tom Harlow, Jeremy Troutman, Jennifer Hawkins, Carlos Salina, Jason Russell, and Derek Trambaugh. Their willingness to participate and have fun while helping us with this project made it an enjoyable experience for all. Many thanks also to Ryan Rudd, our photographer who shot 282 different photos over a two-day period. Few cameramen have Ryan's patience and perseverance to get the job done. Finally, we owe a big thanks to Dr. Jim Peterson. His passion for producing professional educational materials to better the industry helps motivate us to create these materials. Thanks Jim for believing in us!

Contents

Having each been involved with the fitness industry for over 25 years, we have come to realize the importance of "perspective." In reality, our industry is a relatively new industry that has grown by leaps and bounds as commercial organizations have brought new exercise machines to the marketplace, designed a seemingly endless array of exercise and fitness-related devices and equipment, and developed new programs that purport to address the various fitness concerns of the public.

Given the ever-changing number and nature of fitness tools and exercise options available to fitness professionals, a critical issue has arisen—How should all of these things be best used in combination? In response to this concern, we developed the progressive functional system to help fitness professionals address this question. Part of the reason that we developed this new system was the fact that we saw many group exercise instructors and personal trainers using only the commercial fitness equipment that "they" preferred. We also observed new fads and trends that arrived and seemed to "take over" the market, but were not suitable exercises for the mainstream.

Since so many equipment and exercise choices exist, a system of analysis to help instructors identify the most effective, safe, and appropriate exercises for their individual clients and/or classes is needed. As a result, we designed the progressive functional training system to provide both fitness professionals and health professionals with an appropriate way to analyze exercises and select those exercises that will enhance the health and well-being of all participants. In time, you will discover that this system is an exceptional, practical tool for selecting the exercises that the individuals with whom you are working need. In addition, we have added a CD-ROM of all the pictures in the book to help you give your clients a visual image of the exercises on one sheet of paper. When we first put this book out, we saw trainers copying the pages and cutting and pasting exercises on a sheet of paper for their clients. The initial intent of this book was to educate fitness professionals—now we are expanding the concept to the consumer. The following pages offer specific instructions for how to use the CD-ROM.

We hope you enjoy learning this new system and using the CD-ROM to share it with your clients/participants. We also hope you make this progression an integral part of your professional efforts and practice. If it enhances your ability to have a positive impact on the fitness level of others, then the effort involved in developing this system and writing this book will have been worthwhile.

Preface

HOW TO USE THE CD-ROM

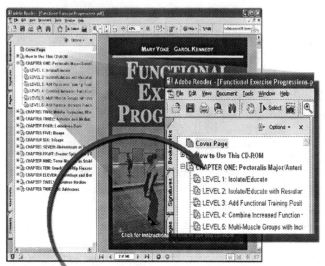

You can select a chapter using the "Bookmarks" panel on the left-hand portion of the screen.

You can also directly access a "Level" within your chosen chapter by clicking the "down" arrow.

After choosing a chapter you may also access a "Level" within the chosen chapter from the chapter title page.

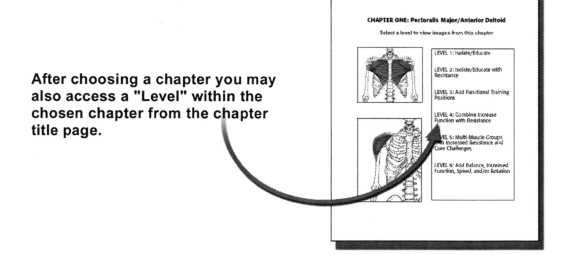

HOW TO USE THE CD-ROM
(Continued)

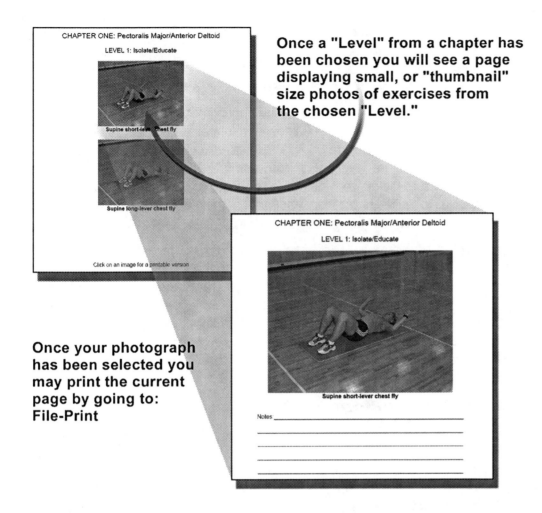

Once a "Level" from a chapter has been chosen you will see a page displaying small, or "thumbnail" size photos of exercises from the chosen "Level."

Once your photograph has been selected you may print the current page by going to: File-Print

The controls at the bottom center of the screen add additional navigational features

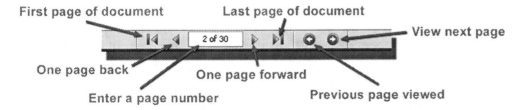

First page of document

Last page of document

View next page

One page back

One page forward

Previous page viewed

Enter a page number

Utilizing the functional exercise progression concept outlined in this book can help you become a more skilled fitness professional. The book presents thirteen sample progressions: six for the upper body, three for the torso, and four for the lower body. All of the exercises in each progression are illustrated and the key alignment issues are described, in order to make this book as user-friendly as possible.

Most fitness professionals are familiar with approximately 1-4 different exercises for each major muscle group. But, did you know that in reality, each group has at least 20-40 exercises? This book includes 17-23 exercises for each major muscle group, arranged according to the level of difficulty—progressing from easiest to the most difficult to perform. All factors considered, the ultimate goal for individuals who perform the exercises is to have them progress through the continuum towards increased function in activities of daily living.

As a fitness professional, it is beneficial for you to have a large repertoire of exercises in your "toolbox". This will help you in a variety of ways, for example, to select the most appropriate exercise for each client if you're a personal trainer, or the best exercises for your class, if you're a group fitness leader. Even when leading a class, instructors must be able to individualize "on the spot" and adjust the exercises according to each participant's needs. Knowing a large number of exercises and being able to appropriately apply them for each client and/or class is one of the hallmarks of a skilled and well-qualified fitness professional.

What is an Exercise Progression?

The term "progression", used in the traditional sense, refers to gradually overloading the body's systems (i.e., increasing the training stimulus over time) to incrementally expose the body to ever higher levels of physiological stress. The body, in turn, responds to these demands by achieving specific fitness adaptations. With resistance training, for example, the muscles gradually and appropriately become stronger and develop a higher level of endurance, as well as achieve an enhanced level of neuromuscular control, coordination, and balance.

As with all forms of physical activity, a sound progression can be achieved by appropriately manipulating the variables of frequency, intensity, duration, and/or mode of exercise. This book addresses the last variable—the mode (type) of exercise.

As such, a key issue arises concerning how the mode or the specific exercises can be progressed to place a gradual and appropriate overload on the bodily systems involved in order to enhance the individual's level of fitness.

In response to this factor, we have devised a method of categorizing exercises that helps quantify progression with regard to mode or type. Each of the progressions presented in this text includes a recommended order of exercises that progresses from easiest to hardest, utilizing the following exercise continuum:

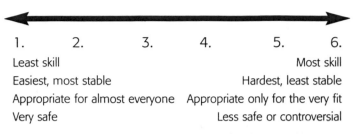

1.	2.	3.	4.	5.	6.

Least skill   Most skill

Easiest, most stable   Hardest, least stable

Appropriate for almost everyone   Appropriate only for the very fit

Very safe   Less safe or controversial

"Less skilled" exercises require less balance, stability, proprioceptive activity, and motor control. As a general rule, these exercises are safer for almost everyone and require the least amount of cueing on the part of the instructor. At the other end of the continuum are exercises that need a great deal of skill and require an ability to maintain joint integrity, including the joints of the spine, a factor that is commonly referred to as core stability. Core stability is the ability to maintain the neck, spine, scapulae, and pelvis in their ideal alignment, no matter how difficult the exercise.

The most difficult exercises also place a high demand on the body's proprioceptors and on the neuromuscular system for smooth coordination. As a result, the ability to perform challenging exercises safely depends on the exerciser's specific skills and overall fitness level. Many sport-specific exercises are at this end of the continuum. Examples of difficult and controversial exercises include: dead lifts, plyometric lunges, handstand shoulder presses, and V-sits. Although these exercises are usually considered as being very difficult to perform and as having a higher risk of injury, a very fit person with excellent skill, fitness, and core stability might actually be able to perform them safely and appropriately. These difficult exercises are not necessarily "better" or "worse" than exercises at the left end of the continuum. The highly challenging exercises suggested in this book at the end of each progression are simply options for those few skilled individuals who are in competitive athletics or who may want variety and the ultimate challenge in their workouts. The key issue here is appropriateness. Fitness professionals and exercisers must select exercises that are appropriate for their needs and fitness levels, always keeping safety in mind.

What is a *Functional* Exercise Progression?

In functional training, the muscles are trained and developed in such a way as to make the performance of everyday activities easier, smoother, safer, and more efficient. Functional exercises improve your ability to function independently in the real world. This factor underlies what is perhaps the most important benefit of exercising regularly—everyday activities become easier and a person's quality of life improves as the individual's level of fitness increases. Accordingly, the functional exercise progressions explained and illustrated in this book are designed to produce enhanced everyday function, both for the general population, and, in several examples, for those individuals involved in sport-specific activities.

How Does the Functional Exercise Progression System Work?

The functional exercise progression system has been organized into six levels, progressing from easiest to hardest:

■ Level #1—*isolate/educate*

At this initial level, the individual's focus is on muscle isolation, allowing the exerciser to learn to selectively contract individual muscles or muscle groups. As a result, exercisers gain confidence as their level of body awareness and knowledge of muscle functions increase.

Exercises shown at this level are usually performed in the supine or prone position, with as much of the body in contact with the floor or bench as possible, thereby lessening the need for stabilizer muscle involvement. As a result, these exercises are generally quite safe; just about everyone can learn to do them effectively with minimal risk of injury. To enhance the participant's muscle awareness and knowledge of how the body works, gravity is usually the only form of resistance applied when performing exercises at this level.

■ Level #2—*isolate/educate: add resistance*

At this level, external resistance is added with machines, weights, increased lever length, or elastic bands and tubes, while keeping the stabilizer involvement to a minimum. In many cases, the actual exercise is the same as in level #1. It should be noted that for both level #1 and level #2, safety and alignment cueing on the part of the instructor is minimized. All factors considered, it's relatively easy to get exercisers to perform these types of exercises safely and effectively, while maintaining proper form.

■ Level #3—*add functional training positions*

At this level, the type of exercise given is usually performed while seated or standing, both of which are more functional positions for most individuals. By moving to seated or standing positions, the exerciser's base of support is reduced, thereby increasing the challenge of utilizing the stabilizing muscles effectively during the exercise. In most progressions, the targeted muscle group is still isolated as a primary mover.

■ Level #4—*combine increasing function with resistance*

At this level, resistance from gravity, external weights, machines, and/or bands and tubes is maximized, while applying increased overload to the core stabilizer muscles in functional positions.

■ Level #5—*multi-muscle groups with increased resistance and core challenge*

At this level, multiple muscle groups and joint actions are employed in each exercise simultaneously. The demands placed on muscular fitness, balance, coordination, and torso stability are progressed to an even greater degree.

■ Level #6—*add balance, increased functional challenge, speed, and/or rotational movements*

At this level, the exercises may require balancing on one leg, using a wobble board or stability ball, adding plyometric movements, incorporating spinal rotation while lifting, or some other creative or sport-specific maneuver. Because the potential risk of injury is increased, instructors should be cautious and prudent. Fitness professionals should keep in mind that many clients, depending on each individual's health history, fitness level, and level of motivation, will never be able to perform some of the exercises at this level.

Safety First

In order to minimize the risk of injury or any adverse health-related event from occurring, fitness professionals should keep the following points in mind when working with clients:

- Instructors must always perform a health-risk screening and a fitness assessment on those with whom they are working. If a client or student has any health issues or history of previous injury, an appropriate medical clearance should be obtained, according to ACSM guidelines.

- Before progressing to a higher level on the continuum, clients and/or students should be able to perform all given exercises up to that point with correct form and alignment for the duration of the exercise set.

- Instructors must be ready to modify any exercise, if required, to enhance safety. This step may involve showing a completely different exercise from an earlier point on the continuum.

- Instructors must always consider the ratio of benefit to risk. They should ask themselves whether the benefit of performing a level #6-type of exercise outweighs the potential risk for a particular client. Remember, it is not always necessary or even desirable for some exercisers to move to levels #5 or #6, where many of the suggested exercises will not be appropriate for all individuals.

Summary Points

It is our hope that by reading this book, you will gain new ideas for exercise programming and will have at your disposal a potential evaluation process that you can utilize to select the "best" exercises for those with whom you are working. Furthermore, we hope that this selection system can serve as a handy way for you to view and categorize the exercises in your own exercise "toolbox". We challenge you to come up with some additional progressions of your own, or utilize the progression concept detailed in this book at an inservice at your facility to help other instructors improve their abilities to share the exceptional benefits of exercise with clients and/or students.

PART ONE: UPPER BODY PROGRESSIONS

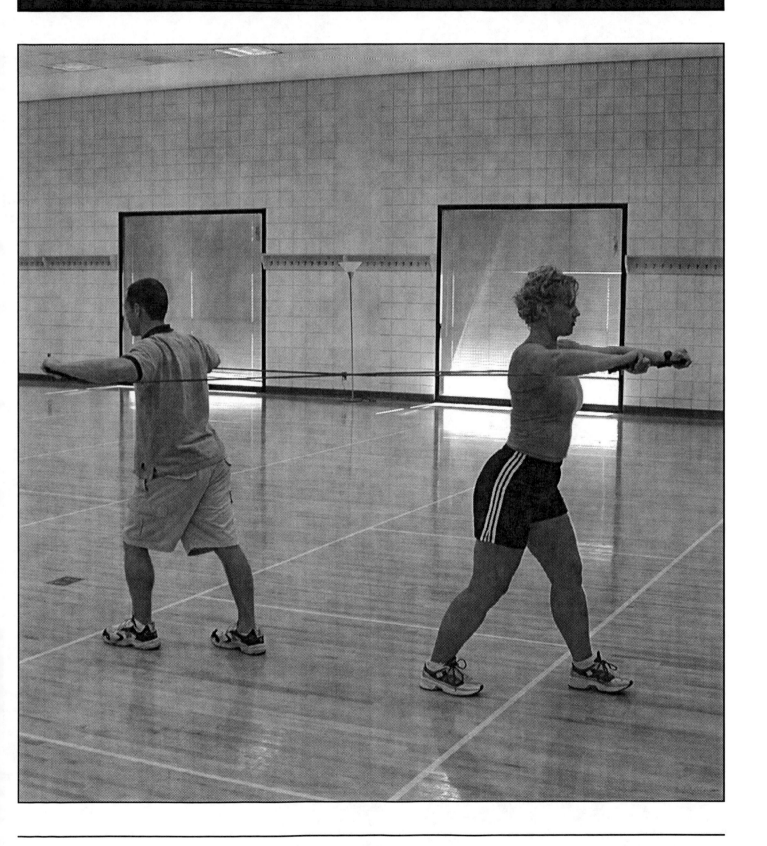

CHAPTER ONE
Pectoralis Major/Anterior Deltoid

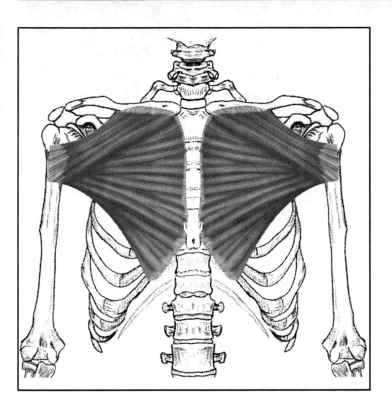

PECTORALIS MAJOR

Primary Joint Actions:

- Shoulder flexion (clavicular portion)
- Shoulder horizontal adduction (both parts)
- Shoulder adduction (sternal portion)
- Shoulder extension (sternal portion)

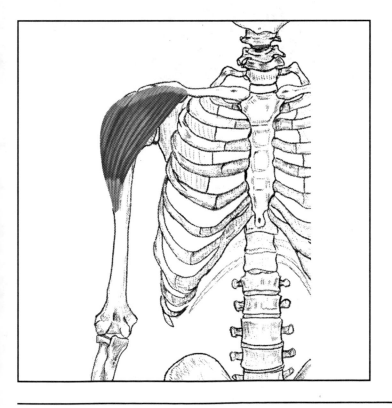

ANTERIOR DELTOID

Primary Joint Actions:

- Shoulder flexion
- Shoulder horizontal adduction

Note: As a general guideline, the exerciser should exhale on the concentric (shortening) phase of the movement.

LEVEL 1: Isolate/Educate

■ **1-1a. Supine short lever chest fly:**

Lie on the back with the knees bent, and the spine, neck, and scapulae in neutral. Start with the shoulders flexed at 90° (upper arms vertical) and the elbows bent. Smoothly open and lower the arms, keeping the elbows bent. Return to the starting position, engaging the chest muscles.

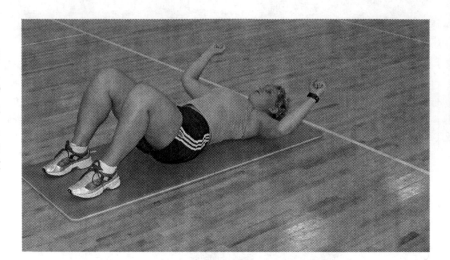

■ **1-2b. Supine long-lever chest fly:**

Lie on the back with the knees bent, and the spine, neck, and scapulae in neutral. Start with the shoulders flexed at 90° (arms long and vertical) and the elbows softly curved. Smoothly open and lower the arms, keeping the elbows still. Return to the starting position, contracting the chest muscles throughout.

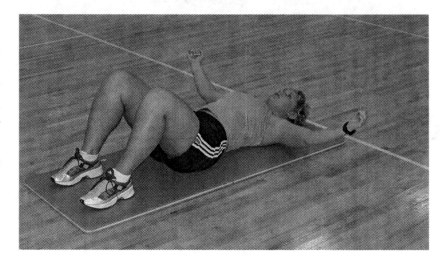

LEVEL 2: Isolate/Educate with Resistance

■ **1-2a. Supine short-lever fly with weights:**

Lie on the back on the bench with the knees bent, and the spine, neck, and scapulae in neutral. Start with the shoulders flexed at 90° (upper arms vertical) and the elbows bent. Smoothly open and lower the arms, keeping the elbows bent. Return to the starting position, engaging the chest muscles. Avoid opening the arms too wide.

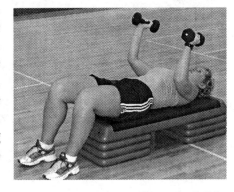

■ **1-2b. Seated pec dec on the Badger variable resistance VR machine:**

Sit with the spine, neck, and scapulae in neutral. Maintaining the shoulder blades against the pad, bring the arms towards each other, contracting the chest muscles. Avoid opening the arms too wide and increasing the risk of injury to the shoulder joint.

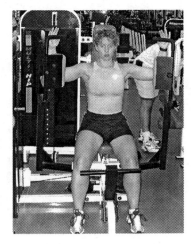

■ **1-2c. Incline chest fly with weights:**

Lie on the back on an incline bench (the greater the incline, the greater the recruitment of the deltoid muscles), with both feet on the floor, the abdominals contracted, and the spine, neck,

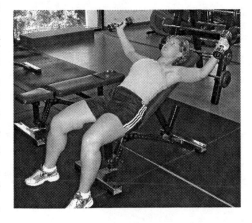

and scapulae in neutral. Start with the arms vertical and perpendicular to the floor, with the elbows slightly flexed. Under control, slowly lower the weights until the upper arms are level with the chest; return to the starting position, engaging the chest muscles. Avoid excessive range of motion. Keep the elbows and wrists still.

■ **1-2d. Seated unilateral pec dec on the Paramount variable resistance VR machine:**

Sit with the spine, neck, and scapulae in neutral. Maintaining the shoulder blades against the pad, bring one arm at a time towards the center, contracting the chest muscles. Maintain stability on the non-working side; keep the shoulders level. Avoid opening the arms too wide.

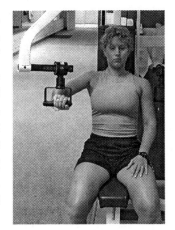

■ **1-2e. Bench press at Smith machine with spotter:**

Lie supine on the bench, adjusting the foot placement so that the spine is maintained in neutral. The bar should be aligned directly above the chest muscles. Using a wide, pronated grip with the upper arm angled 80°-90° out from the torso, slowly lower the bar. Press up, engaging the chest muscles. Avoid hyperextending the elbows.

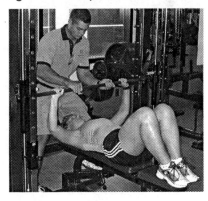

LEVEL 3: Add Functional Training Positions

■ **1-3a. Standing chest press with tubing and partner:**

Interlock the tubes and face away from partner, stepping away for optimal resistance. Hold the handles in front of the shoulders, with the tubes under the arms. Stagger feet and maintain a long line from the back heel to the head. Engage abdominals and keep the spine, neck, pelvis, and scapulae in neutral. Both partners press out at chest height simultaneously.

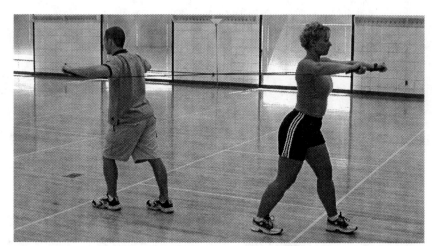

■ **1-3b. Supine chest fly on stability ball:**

Lie on the back with the shoulder blades, neck, and head on the ball. Maintain a planked, level position with the entire lower body, buttocks and abdominals contracted. Start with the shoulders flexed at 90° (arms vertical) and the elbows slightly bent. Smoothly open and lower the arms, keeping the elbows stable. Return to the starting position, engaging the chest muscles. The difficulty level of the exercise may be increased by bringing the feet together.

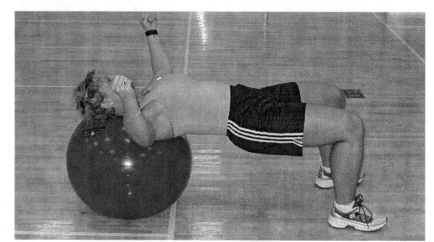

LEVEL 4: Combine Increased Function with Resistance

■ **1-4a. Seated cable crossover:**

Sit on the bench without back support, keeping the spine, neck, and scapulae stabilized in neutral. Perform a fly movement, bringing the handles towards each other in front of the chest, while contracting the chest muscles. Control the lengthening phase and avoid an excessive range of motion. Keep the shoulders down and away from the ears.

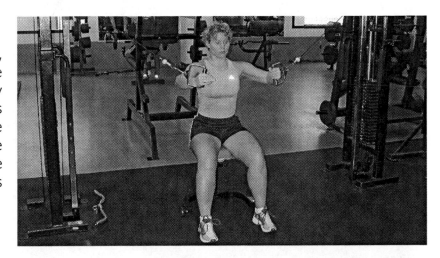

■ **1-4b. Bilateral chest fly on a Free Motion VR machine:**

Stand facing away from the machine (cable crossover with high pulleys). Stagger the feet, and maintain one long line from the back heel through the head. Keep the knees soft, the abdominals contracted, the spine, neck, and scapulae in neutral, and the elbows slightly flexed. Bring the handles towards each other in front of the chest and control the lengthening phase, avoiding an excessive range of motion.

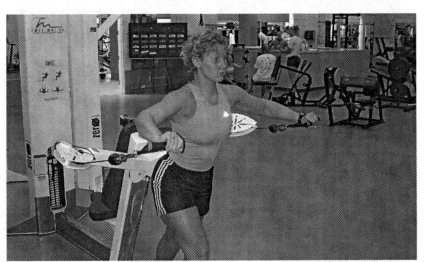

■ **1-4c. Unilateral chest fly on a Free Motion VR machine:**

Stand facing away from the machine (cable crossover with high pulleys). Stagger the feet, and maintain one long line from the back heel through the head. Keep the knees soft, the abdominals contracted, the spine, neck, and scapulae in neutral, and the elbows slightly flexed. Bring one handle at a time towards the center, stabilizing the other side. Keep the shoulders level, and avoid twisting the spine.

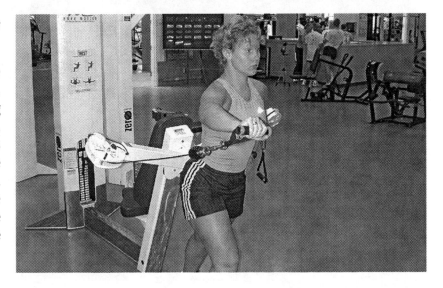

LEVEL 5: Multi-Muscle Groups with Increased Resistance and Core Challenge

■ **1-5a. Alternating lunges with chest press:**

Anchor the tubing to the wall and grasp the handles, keeping the tubing under the arms. Face away from the wall. Lunge forward, while simultaneously performing a chest press. Repeat on the other side. Maintain a neutral pelvis, spine, neck, and scapulae, keeping the torso upright. When lunging forward, the front knee should flex no deeper than 90°.

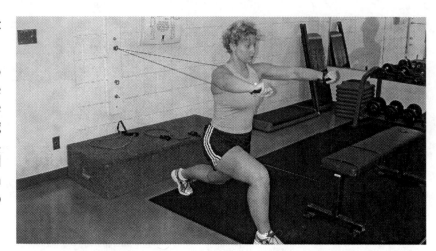

■ **1-5b. Push-up series:**

For optimal pectoralis major and anterior deltoid recruitment, keep the shoulders abducted 80°-90° away from the torso. In all push-ups, the spine and neck should be stabilized, with the abdominals contracted. The scapulae should remain depressed and mid-way between protraction and retraction. Exhale when pushing up. The following variations of push-ups can be performed (shown with increasing levels of difficulty):

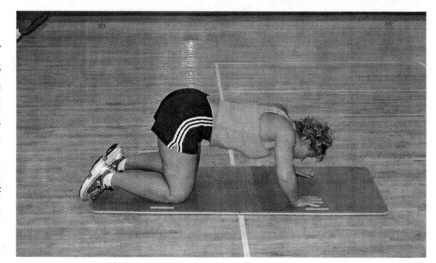

→ **Table top push-up**

Hinge the hips at a right angle while on the hands and knees. Lower the top of the forehead to the floor, keeping the neck in a straight line with the spine.

→ **Regular knee push-up**

While on the hands and knees, form one long line (modified plank) from the knees through the head. Lower the chest and nose towards the floor, maintaining a stable plank throughout.

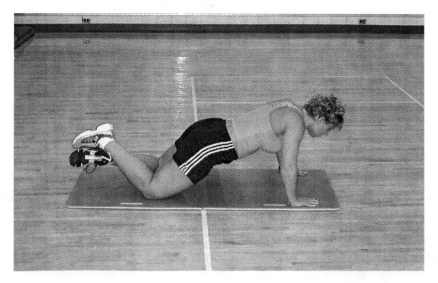

LEVEL 5: Multi-Muscle Groups with Increased Resistance and Core Challenge (cont'd)

→ **Full push-up**

Maintain a long line from the heels to the head, keeping the entire body in a plank position and in neutral.

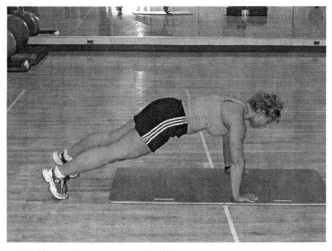

→ **Full push-up on one foot**

Maintain a long line from the heels to the head, keeping the entire body in a plank position and in neutral. Perform push-ups while balanced on one foot, with the other leg in the air.

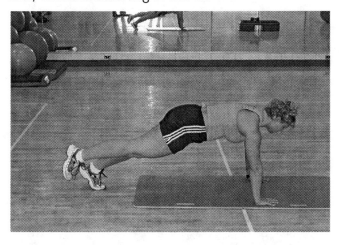

→ **Push-up with stability ball under knees**

Lying prone on a ball, walk-out to the push-up position, with the ball under the thighs or the knees. Keep the abdominals securely contracted.

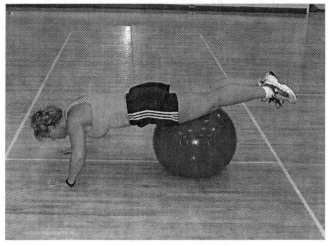

→ **Push-up with stability ball under feet**

Lying prone on a ball, walk-out to the push-up position, with the ball under the shoelaces or the toes. Maintain a secure plank, with the buttocks and abdominals contracted while pushing up, and the neck in neutral. To increase the difficulty level of the exercise, perform with just one foot on the ball, with the other leg lifted.

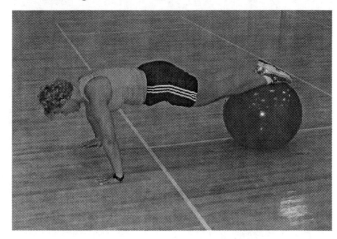

LEVEL 6: Add Balance, Increase Function, Speed, and/or Rotation

■ **1-6a. Push-up with stability ball, alternating with tuck:**

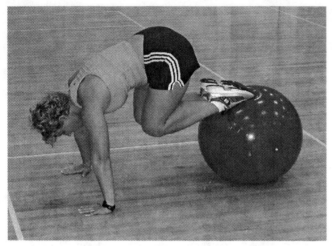

Lying prone on a ball, walk-out to the push-up position, with the ball under the shoelaces. Maintain a secure plank, with the buttocks and abdominals contracted while pushing up, and the neck in neutral. After each push-up, perform a "tuck"—flex the knees and hips, while drawing the ball in under the shins. Straighten the knees and hips, and push-up.

■ **1-6b. Push-up alternated with side plank:**

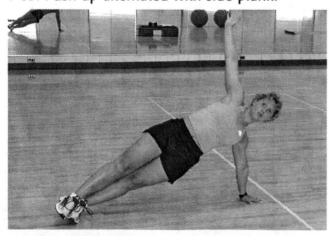

Perform a full push-up on the floor. After pushing up, move directly into a side plank, with the weight on one hand and the feet stacked. Pause and balance, and then return back to both hands and push-up as before. Alternate sides, keeping the pelvis, spine, neck, and scapulae in neutral, and the abdominals contracted.

■ **1-6c. Push-up on slideboard:**

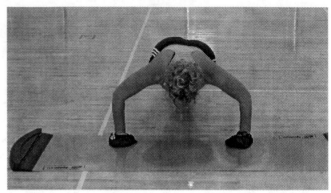

The exercise may be performed on either the knees (modified) or the toes (full). Place the slide booties on the hands, and the hands on the slide under the shoulders, and get in the push-up position. Slowly slide both hands laterally away from each other, while descending in the push-up. Using the chest muscles, slide the hands back in towards the starting position under the shoulders, while pushing up. Maintain the pelvis, spine, neck, and scapulae in neutral, while keeping the abdominals contracted. Avoid an excessive range of motion on the descent.

■ **1-6d. Martial arts unilateral hook with hip rotation using a Free Motion machine:**

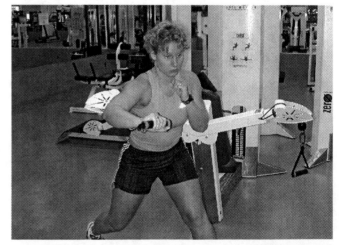

Adjust the pulley to the "mid"-position just below the shoulder. Grasping the handle, perform a boxers hook move, while incorporating a hip rotation. Keep the abdominals contracted, and the pelvis, spine, and neck in neutral.

CHAPTER TWO
Middle Trapezius, Rhomboids, and Posterior Deltoid

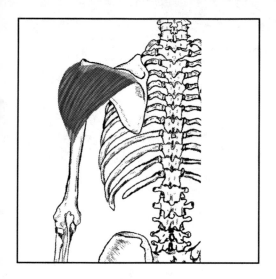

POSTERIOR DELTOID

Primary Joint Actions:

- Shoulder horizontal abduction
- Shoulder extension

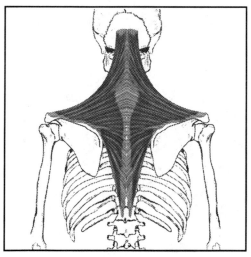

TRAPEZIUS

Primary Joint Actions:

- Trapezius I
  - √ Scapular elevation
- Trapezius II
  - √ Scapular elevation
  - √ Scapular upward rotation

- Trapezius III
  - √ Scapular retraction
- Trapezius IV
  - √ Scapular depression
  - √ Scapular upward rotation

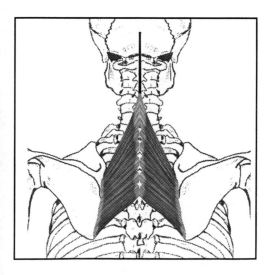

RHOMBOIDS

Primary Joint Actions:

- Scapular retraction
- Scapular elevation
- Scapular downward rotation

Note: The aforementioned muscles have an important role in helping to counteract the effects of chest work and in helping to maintain proper posture.

LEVEL 1: Isolate/Educate

■ **2-1a. Prone short-lever reverse flys (dorsal lifts):**

Lie prone, face down, with the neck, spine, and pelvis in neutral, and the abdominals engaged. Place the arms at a 90° angle to the torso, flex the elbows at a 90° angle. Retract the scapulae, while lifting the arms from the floor. Contract the middle trapezius and rhomboids.

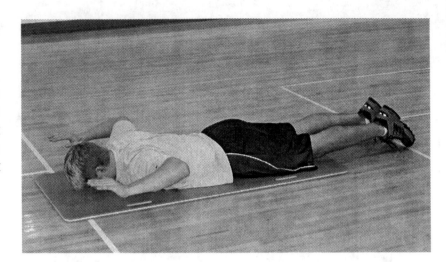

■ **2-1b. Prone long-lever reverse flys:**

Lie prone, face down, with the neck, spine, and pelvis in neutral, and the abdominals engaged. Place the arms at a 90° level to the torso. Retract the scapulae, lifting the arms from the floor.

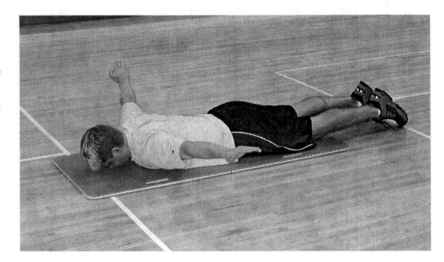

LEVEL 2: Isolate/Educate with Resistance

■ **2-2a. Badger reverse fly VR machine:**

Sit with the torso stabilized against the pad, with the spine and neck in neutral. Contract the middle trapezius and rhomboids and retract (adduct) the shoulder blades. Avoid arching the lower back.

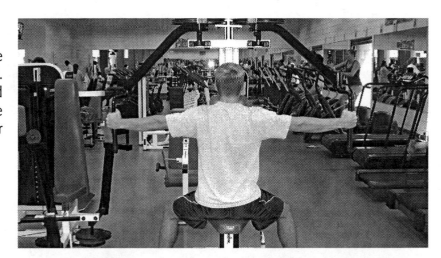

■ **2-2b. Paramount fly VR machine unilateral option:**

Sit with the torso stabilized against the pad, and the spine and neck in neutral. Contract the middle traps and rhomboids and retract (adduct) the shoulder blade on one side. Avoid arching the back. Repeat on the other side.

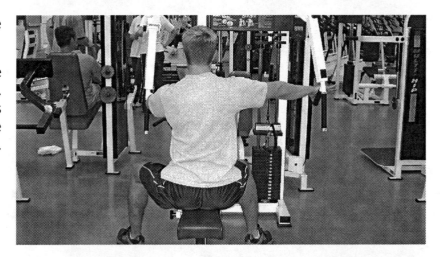

■ **2-2c. Reverse flys on bench with dumbbells:**

Lie prone on a bench with the abdominals contracted and the ribs and hips in contact with the pad. Keeping the arms perpendicular to the torso, retract the scapulae, lifting the arms. Contract the posterior deltoids as well as the scapular retractors (mid-traps and rhomboids).

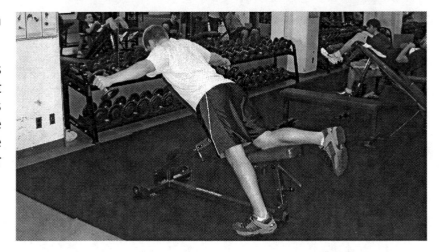

LEVEL 3: Add Functional Training Positions

■ **2-3a. Standing retraction with band/tube:**

Stand with the knees soft, the pelvis, spine, and neck in neutral, and the abdominals contracted. Hold a band or a tube in front of the chest with the elbows up and the scapulae depressed. Perform a short range of motion high row, retracting the shoulder blades.

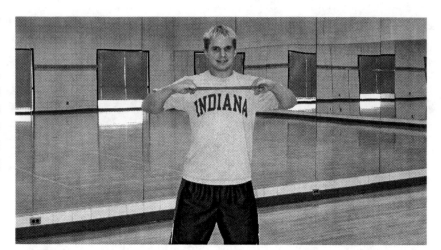

■ **2-3b. Seated high row with tube:**

Sit with the legs in front of the body, with the knees slightly flexed. Maintain the spine and neck in neutral, sitting on a pad if necessary. Wrap tubing around the soles of the feet, crossing the tube. Perform a high (horizontal) row with the palms down, the elbows up, and the shoulders abducted at an 80°-90° angle to the body. Keep the scapulae depressed while performing retraction.

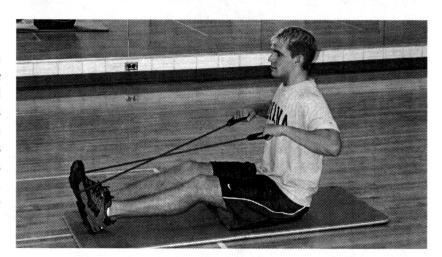

■ **2-3c. Prone short-lever reverse fly on a stability ball:**

Lie prone with a stability ball under the abdomen. Maintain a long, planked line from the heels to the head. Keeping the neck, spine, and pelvis in neutral, place the arms at 90° to torso, and flex the elbows at 90°. Retract the scapulae and contract the middle trapezius, rhomboids, and posterior deltoids.

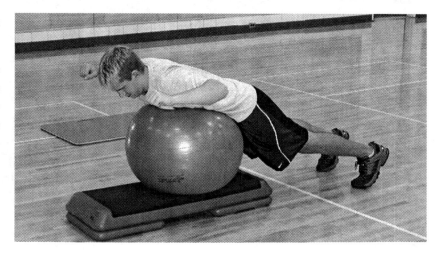

LEVEL 4: Combine Increased Function with Resistance

■ **2-4a. AFS seated high row at the low pulley:**

Sit with the spine and neck in neutral, with the knees slightly flexed, and the abdominals contracted. Grasp the short, straight bar with a pronated (palms down) grip. Perform a high 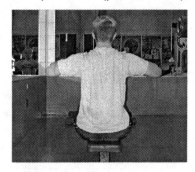 (horizontal) row with the elbows lifted and the shoulders abducted at an 80°-90° angle to the body. Keep the scapulae depressed while performing retraction.

■ **2-4b. Standing high row with partner using tubing:**

Stand facing the partner, with the tubes interlocked. Step away to the desired level of resistance. Keep the knees soft, the abdominals in, the pelvis, spine, and neck in neutral, 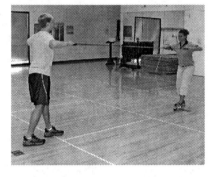 and the scapulae down. Perform a high (horizontal) row with the palms down, the elbows up, and the shoulders abducted at an 80°-90° angle to body.

■ **2-4c. Prone reverse flys on a stability ball with weights:**

Lie prone with the stability ball under the abdomen. Maintain a long, planked line from the heels to the head. Keeping the neck, spine, and pelvis in neutral, place the arms at a 90° angle to the torso, and keep the elbows slightly bent. Hold 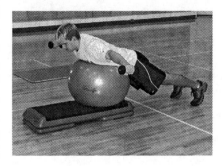 weights with palms down. Retract scapulae and contract middle trapezius, rhomboids, and posterior deltoids.

■ **2-4d. Standing reverse cable cross-over:**

Stand between the high pulleys with the knees soft, the abdominals contracted, and the pelvis, spine, and neck in neutral. Grasp the pulley handle on the left side with the 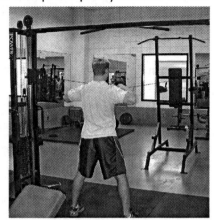 right hand; grasp the pulley handle on the right side with the left hand. (The arms will be crossed in front of the chest). Perform a high-row type movement with the elbows lifted and the shoulders abducted at a 80°-90° angle to the body. Keep the scapulae depressed while performing retraction.

■ **2-4e. Bent-over unilateral reverse fly with low pulley:**

Stand with parallel feet, shoulder-width apart near the low pulley unit. Bend over in a hip hinge and place the non-working hand on the thigh for support. Engage the abdominals and keep the spine and neck neutral. Grasping the 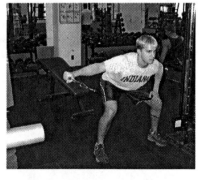 handle, perform a unilateral reverse fly, keeping the elbow slightly flexed, the wrist straight, and the shoulders still and level. Move through the fly into a unilateral scapular retraction.

LEVEL 5: Multi-Muscle Groups with Increased Resistance and Core Challenge

■ **2-5a. 4-count bilateral bent-over row:**

With the feet parallel and shoulder-width apart, hinge at the hips and place the spine and neck in neutral, with the abdominals contracted. Perform a high row in four counts: 1) row, bringing the elbows up, 2) retract the scapulae, 3) release the scapulae, and 4) return to the starting position. Engage the mid-trapezius, rhomboids, and posterior deltoids.

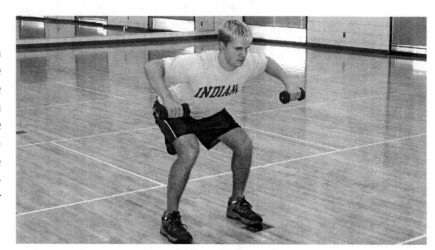

■ **2-5b. 4-count bilateral bent-over row with external rotation:**

With the feet parallel and shoulder-width apart, hinge at the hips and place the spine and neck in neutral, with the abdominals contracted. Perform the exercise in four counts: 1) row, bringing the elbows up, 2) externally rotate the shoulders (the palms face the floor), 3) de-rotate the shoulders back to the row position, and 4) return to the starting position. This exercise incorporates the shoulder external rotator cuff muscles (infraspinatus and teres minor).

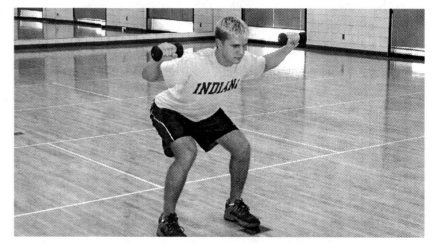

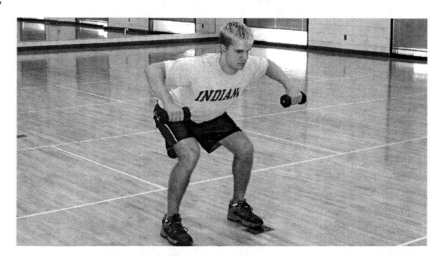

LEVEL 6: Add Balance, Increased Function, Speed, and/or Rotation

■ **2-6a. Alternating front lunges with scapular retraction:**

Have the partner hold and anchor the tubing. While lunging forward and alternating the legs, simultaneously perform a high (horizontal) row with the elbows up and the shoulders abducted at an 80°-90° angle to the body.

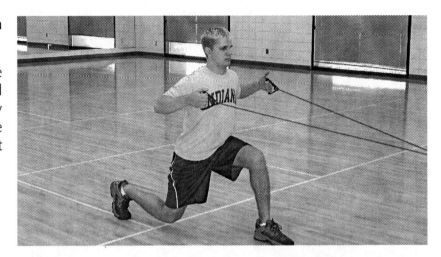

■ **2-6b. Bent-over unilateral high rows on one foot:**

Balancing on one foot, hinge at the hips, keeping the spine and neck neutral, and the abdominals contracted. Start with the arm down. Perform high rows, first with one side, and then the other, alternating feet. Maintain core stability throughout.

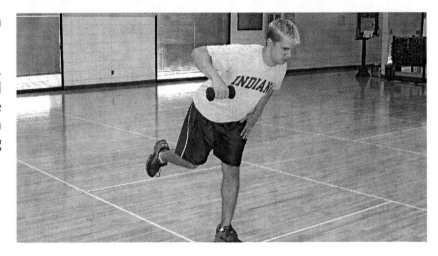

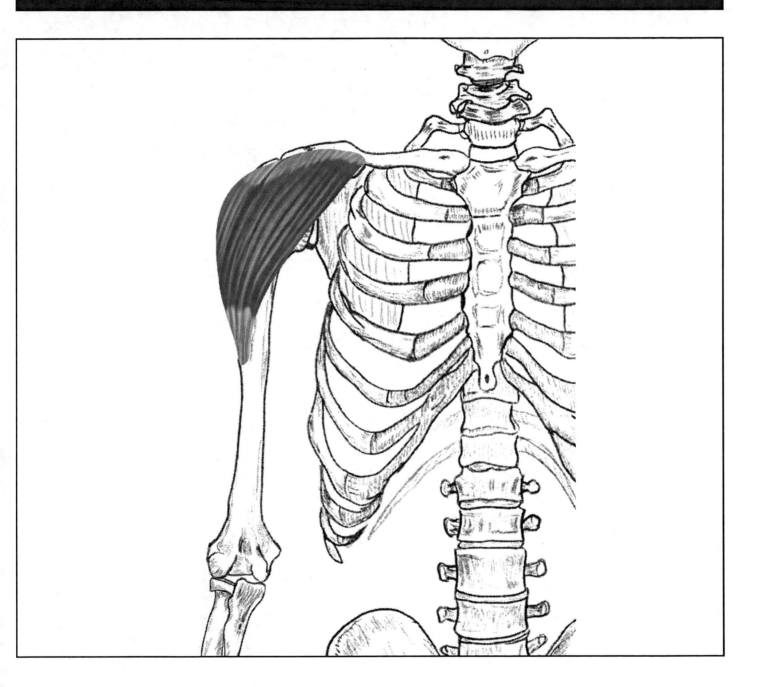

ANTERIOR DELTOID

Primary Joint Actions:

- Shoulder flexion

- Shoulder horizontal adduction

MEDIAL DELTOID

Primary Joint Actions:

- Shoulder abduction

- Shoulder horizontal abduction

LEVEL 1: Isolate/Educate

■ **3-1a. Seated unilateral front raise:**

Sit on a bench with good alignment, with the pelvis, spine, neck and scapulae neutral, and the shoulders level. Slowly perform alternating front raises, contracting the deltoids.

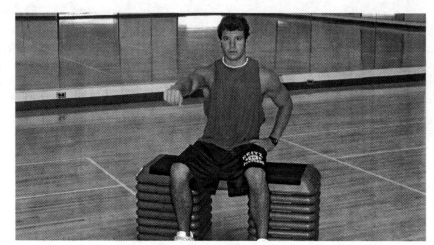

■ **3-1b. Seated bilateral front raise:**

Sit on a bench with good alignment, with the pelvis, spine, neck and scapulae neutral, and the shoulders level. Slowly perform bilateral front raises, contracting the deltoids.

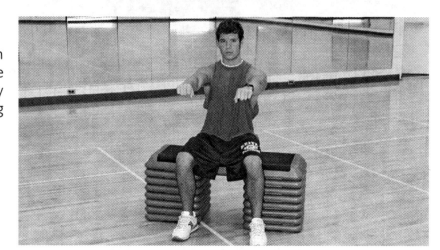

■ **3-1c. Seated lateral raise:**

Sit on a bench with good alignment, with the pelvis, spine, neck, and scapulae neutral, and the shoulders level. Slowly perform lateral raises with the elbows slightly flexed, the wrists neutral, and the palms facing the floor. Abduct the shoulders to no more than a 90° angle to help prevent shoulder impingement.

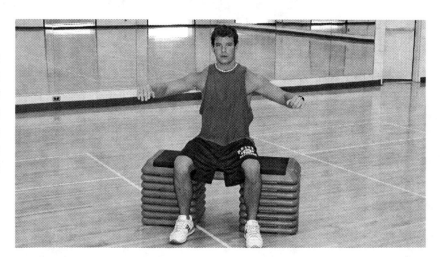

LEVEL 2: Isolate/Educate with Resistance

■ **3-2a. Seated unilateral front raise with dumbbells:**

Sit on a bench with good alignment, with the pelvis, spine, neck, and scapulae neutral, and the shoulders level. Slowly perform alternating front raises with the dumbbells, keeping the wrists straight and contracting the deltoids.

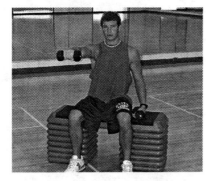

■ **3-2b. Seated bilateral front raise with dumbbells:**

Sit on a bench with good alignment, with the pelvis, spine, neck, and scapulae neutral, and the shoulders level. Slowly perform bilateral front raises with the dumbbells, keeping the wrists straight and contracting the deltoids.

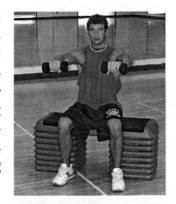

■ **3-2c. Seated lateral raise with dumbbells:**

Sit on a bench with good alignment, with the pelvis, spine, neck, and scapulae neutral, and the shoulders level. Holding dumbbells, slowly perform lateral raises with the elbows slightly flexed, the wrists neutral, and the palms facing the floor. Abduct the shoulders to no more than a 90° angle to help prevent shoulder impingement.

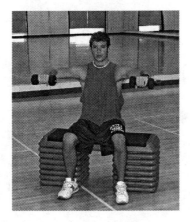

■ **3-2d. Cybex VR machine overhead press:**

Sit at the machine with the pelvis, spine, and neck in neutral; keep the scapulae depressed and the head against the pad. Adjust the seat so that the cam is level with the shoulders. Slowly perform an overhead press, engaging the deltoids.

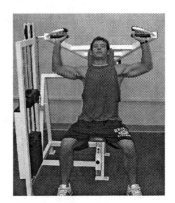

■ **3-2e. Side lying lateral raise on incline bench:**

Lie on the side on an incline bench with the hips and shoulders stacked, and the pelvis, spine, and neck in neutral. Keeping the torso squared, the abdominals contracted, and the scapulae away from the ears, slowly perform a weighted lateral raise with the top arm, keeping the elbow slightly flexed and the wrist in neutral.

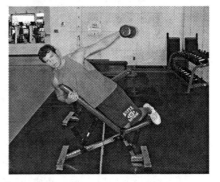

LEVEL 3: Add Functional Training Positions

■ **3-3a. Standing unilateral front raise with tubing:**

Stand in good alignment with a tube anchored under the working-side foot. Keep the knees soft, the pelvis, spine, neck, and scapulae in neutral, and the abdominals contracted. Grasping the handle with the working-side hand, perform a front raise, engaging the deltoids. Maintain a neutral (straight) wrist.

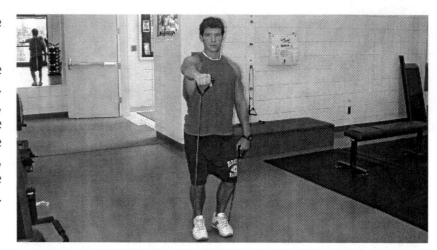

■ **3-3b. Standing lateral raise with tubing:**

Stand in good alignment with a tube anchored under both feet. Keep the knees soft, the pelvis, spine, neck, and scapulae in neutral, and the abdominals contracted. Grasping the handles with both hands, perform lateral raises with the elbows slightly flexed, the wrists neutral, and the palms facing the floor. Abduct the shoulders to no more than a 90° angle to help prevent shoulder impingement.

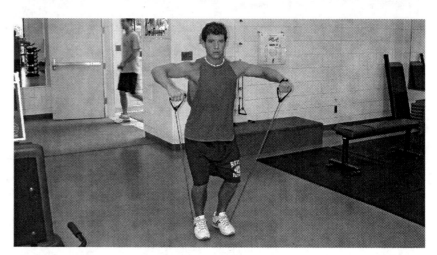

■ **3-3c. Standing overhead press with dumbbells:**

Stand with the knees slightly flexed, the pelvis, spine, and neck in neutral, and the abdominals contracted. Start with the weights level with the shoulders, with the palms facing forwards. Slowly perform an overhead press, keeping the scapulae depressed throughout. Avoid hyperextending the elbows.

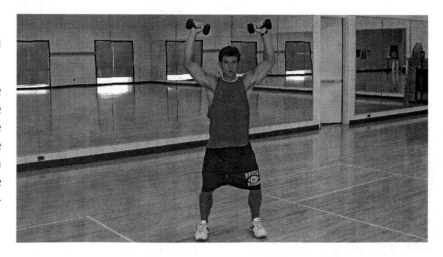

LEVEL 4: Combine Increased Function with Resistance

■ **3-4a. Seated front raise on a stability ball:**

Sit on a stability ball with good alignment, with the pelvis, spine, neck, and scapulae neutral, and the shoulders level. Slowly perform front raises with the dumbbells, keeping the wrists straight and contracting the deltoids. Maintain a stable torso throughout.

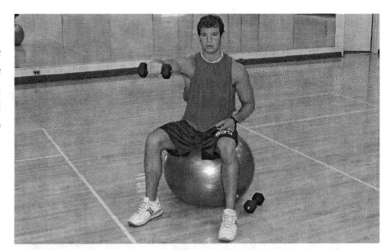

■ **3-4b. Standing upright row at a Smith machine:**

Stand at the Smith machine, with the knees soft, the pelvis, spine, and neck in neutral, and the abdominals contracted. Grasping the bar with a pronated (overhand), narrow grip, perform an upright row. To help avoid shoulder problems, keep the scapulae depressed throughout, and avoid lifting the upper arm greater than 90° of shoulder abduction. Lift with the elbows, not the wrists (keep the wrists neutral). If training for football, wrestling, or bodybuilding, the scapular elevation movement is optional.

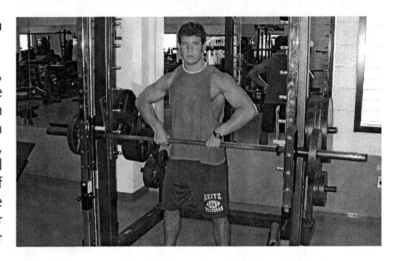

■ **3-4c. Standing one-arm lateral raise at a low pulley:**

Stand sideways to a low pulley, with the knees soft, the pelvis, spine, and neck in neutral, and the abdominals contracted. Grasping the handle with the outside hand, perform a one-armed lateral raise, keeping the elbow slightly bent, the wrist straight, and the scapulae depressed. Engage the deltoids, and maintain squared and level shoulders throughout.

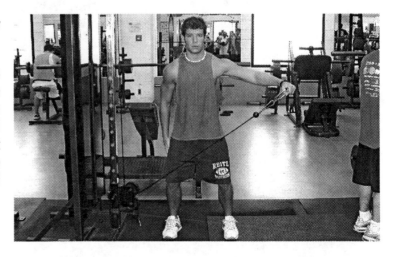

LEVEL 5: Multi-Muscle Groups with Increased Resistance and Core Challenge

■ **3-5a. Overhead press with squat:**

Stand with the knees slightly flexed, the pelvis, spine, and neck in neutral, and the abdominals contracted. Start with the weights level with the shoulders and the palms facing forwards. Slowly perform an overhead press, keeping the scapulae depressed throughout and avoiding hyperextending the elbows. Simultaneously perform a squat, keeping the knees behind the toes and aligned in the direction of the second toe; maintain a neutral spine throughout. Avoid flexing the knees greater than a 90° angle.

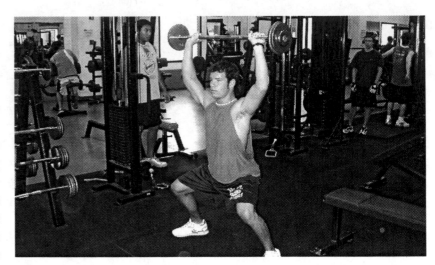

■ **3-5b. Standing lateral raises with hip abduction:**

Stand in a good alignment with the knees soft, the pelvis, spine, neck, and scapulae in neutral, and the abdominals contracted. Holding the dumbbells in both hands, perform lateral raises with the elbows slightly flexed, the wrists neutral, and the palms facing the floor, while simultaneously abducting the leg—first on one side, and then the other. Keep the hips level and the torso still. Abduct the shoulders to no more than a 90° angle to help prevent shoulder impingement.

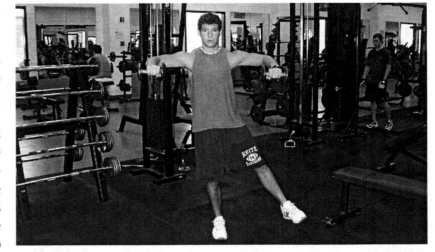

LEVEL 6: Add Balance, Increased Function, Speed, and/or Rotation

■ **3-6a. Seated overhead press on a stability ball, balanced on one foot:**

Sit on a stability ball in good alignment, with the pelvis, spine, and neck in neutral. Hold the dumbbells with the palms facing forwards; balance on one foot, while contracting the abdominals. Slowly perform an overhead press, keeping the scapulae depressed and the torso stable. Avoid hyperextending the elbows.

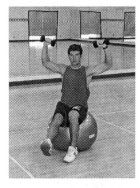

■ **3-6b. Seated unilateral overhead press at the low pulley on a stability ball, balanced on one foot:**

Sit on a stability ball in good alignment, facing away from the low pulley, with the pelvis, spine, and neck in neutral. Grasp the handle on the working side; lift the opposite foot off the floor. Contracting the core muscles and engaging the deltoid, perform a unilateral overhead press, keeping the scapulae depressed.

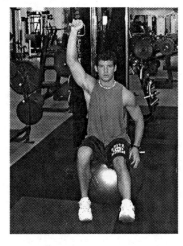

■ **3-6c. Handstand overhead press, with the feet on the wall:**

Stand on the hands, facing the wall, with the feet against the wall, the pelvis, spine, and neck in neutral, and the abdominals contracted. Slowly lower and lift the entire body, performing an overhead press. Engage the deltoids and avoid hyperextending the elbows.

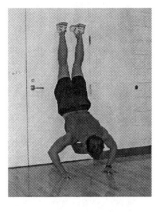

■ **3-6d. Handstand overhead press, piked off a stability ball:**

Roll off the ball into a pike position; dorsiflex the ankles with the toes on the ball. Perform a hip hinge, keeping the spine and neck in neutral, and the abdominals contracted. Slowly lower

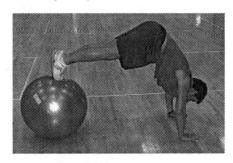

and lift the entire body, performing an overhead press and maintaining core stability. Engage the deltoids and avoid hyperextending the elbows.

■ **3-6e. Handstand overhead press, piked off a stability ball, balanced on one foot.**

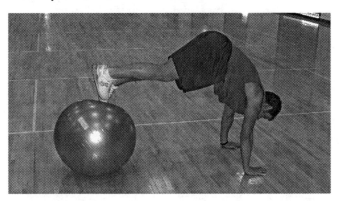

■ **3-6f.** Perform the previous exercise detailed in 3-6d, except raise one foot, making certain to contract the core muscles.

CHAPTER FOUR
Latissimus Dorsi

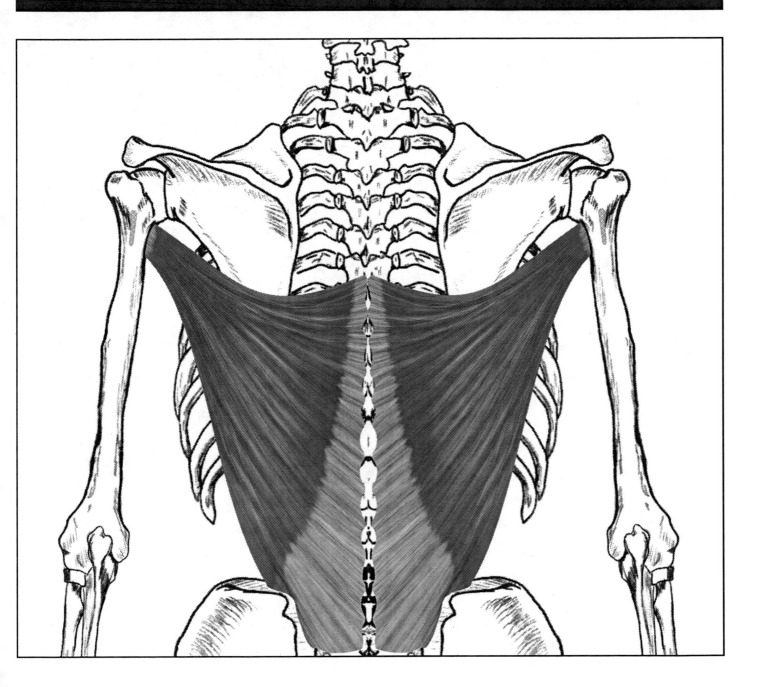

LATISSIMUS DORSI

Primary Joint Actions:

- Shoulder extension
- Shoulder adduction

Assists with shoulder internal rotation and shoulder horizontal abduction.

LEVEL 1: Isolate/Educate

■ **4-1a. Prone shoulder extension on a bench:**

Lie prone on a bench (inclined if necessary to accommodate the length of the arms), with the pelvis, spine, neck, and scapulae in neutral, the abdominals contracted, and the shoulders flexed with the arms hanging vertically. Engaging the lats, perform a bilateral shoulder extension.

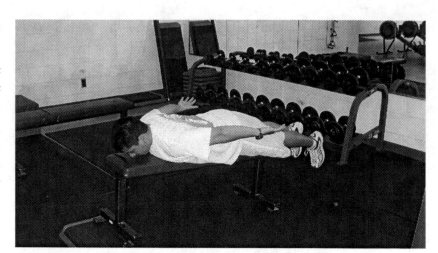

■ **4-1b. Supine pullover on a bench:**

Lie supine on a bench with the feet elevated if necessary to achieve a neutral pelvis, spine, and neck. Start with the shoulders flexed and the arms overhead. Consciously engaging the lats, pull the arms into a vertical position (90° of shoulder flexion).

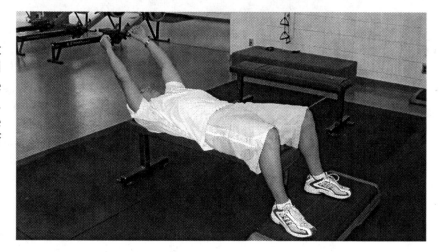

LEVEL 2: Isolate/Educate with Resistance

4-2a. Prone shoulder extension on a bench with dumbbells:

Lie prone on a bench (inclined if necessary to accommodate arm length), with the pelvis, spine, neck, and scapulae in neutral, the abdominals contracted, and the shoulders flexed with the arms hanging vertically. Engaging the lats, perform a bilateral shoulder extension with the weights, keeping the wrists neutral.

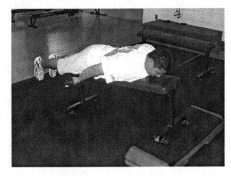

4-2b. Supine pullover on a bench with tubing:

Lie supine on a bench, with the feet elevated if necessary to achieve a neutral pelvis, spine, and neck. Have a partner anchor the tubing. Grasp the handles, with the shoulders flexed and the arms overhead. Consciously engaging the lats, pull the arms into a vertical position (90° of shoulder flexion).

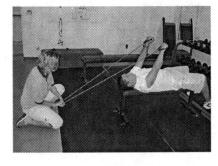

4-2c. Badger lat pullover VR machine:

Adjust the machine so that the cam is level with the shoulder joint; anchor the lower body. Starting with the shoulders flexed and the arms overhead, engage the lats and pull the unit down through the shoulder extension, while exhaling.

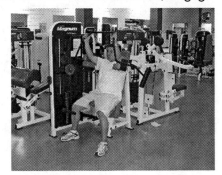

4-2d. AFS seated low row at low pulley:

Sit at a low pulley with the knees slightly flexed, and the spine, neck, and scapulae in neutral. Holding the V bar, contract the lats and perform a low row, keeping the elbows low, while brushing the rib cage with the upper arms. Keep the torso perfectly still throughout.

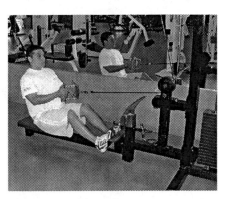

4-2e. Seated lat pulldown:

Sitting at the lat pulldown station (high pulley), keep the spine and neck neutral, the scapulae depressed, and the abdominals contracted. Perform shoulder adduction with a wide grip on the long bar, bringing the bar to the sternum. Keep the torso perfectly still and the scapulae depressed throughout. Avoid the behind-the-neck position because of the increased risk of shoulder-joint injury.

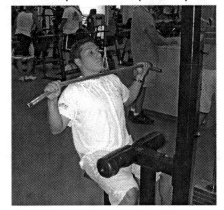

LEVEL 3: Add Functional Training Positions

■ **4-3a. Standing unilateral shoulder extension with a dumbbell:**

Stand with the feet staggered, so that a straight line exists from the back heel to the head. Place the non-working hand on the same-side thigh. Contract the abdominals and maintain the pelvis, spine, neck, and scapulae in neutral. Keep the shoulders squared, while performing shoulder extension, engaging the lats.

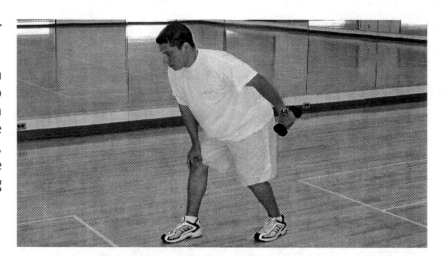

■ **4-3b. Standing alternating pulldown with tubing:**

Stand with the knees soft, the pelvis, spine, and neck in neutral, and the abdominals contracted. Anchor the tubing overhead with the non-moving arm, and grasp the handle on the moving (working) side. Engaging the lats, perform a unilateral pulldown (shoulder adduction), keeping the shoulders and torso still, and maintaining the arms slightly forward of the frontal plane.

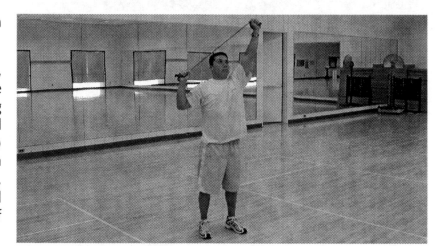

■ **4-3c. Standing bilateral adduction with anchored tubing:**

Anchor the tubing to a hook high on the wall. Grasping the handles, stand with the feet staggered, so that a straight line exists from the back heel to the head, keeping the pelvis, spine, and neck in neutral, and the abdominals contracted. Perform shoulder adduction, contracting the lats and keeping the arms slightly forward of the frontal plane.

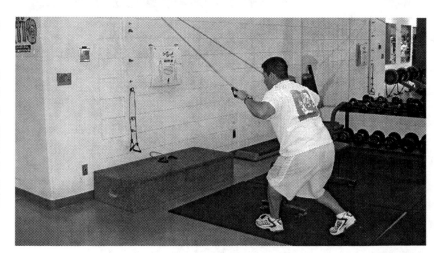

LEVEL 4: Combine Increased Function with Resistance

■ **4-4a. Standing unilateral shoulder extension from a high pulley:**

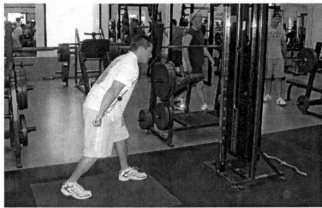

Stand facing a high pulley, with the feet staggered so that a straight line exists from the back heel to the head. Keep the pelvis, spine, and neck in neutral, and the abdominals contracted. Support the non-working hand on the same-side thigh. Grasping the handle with the working hand, perform straight-arm shoulder extension through a full range of motion, engaging the lats and keeping the torso completely still.

■ **4-4b. Prone bilateral shoulder extension on a stability ball with tubing:**

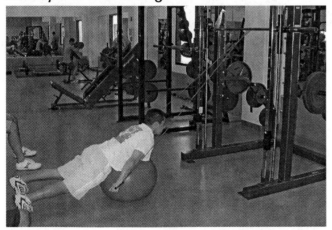

Lie prone on a stability ball with the ball under the abdomen, so that a straight line exists from the heels to the head. Anchor the tubing to a high hook on the wall (or to a high bar on a Smith press) and grasp the handles, starting with the shoulders flexed. Engaging the lats, perform shoulder extension through a full range of motion, while exhaling. Slowly return to the starting position.

■ **4-4c. Paramount VR bilateral seated pulldown:**

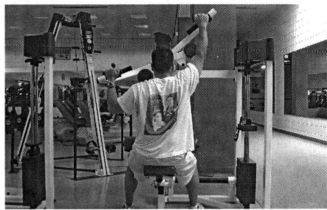

Sit on a bench with a handle in each hand, with the spine and neck in neutral, and the abdominals contracted. Perform a one-arm shoulder adduction, bringing the elbow into the side, while keeping the torso completely still. Repeat on the other side.

■ **4-4d. Free Motion bilateral lat pulldown:**

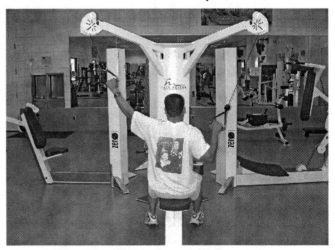

Sit on a bench with a handle in each hand, the spine and neck in neutral, and the abdominals contracted. Perform shoulder adduction, bringing the elbows in to the sides, keeping the torso completely still.

LEVEL 5: Multi-Muscle Groups with Increased Resistance and Core Challenge

■ **4-5a. Stairmaster gravitron pull-ups:**

Kneel on the gravity assisted device, with the pelvis, spine, and neck in neutral, and the abdominals contracted. Using a wide grip, perform shoulder adduction, engaging the lats throughout. A narrow grip (shoulder extension) may be used as a variation. Keep the scapulae depressed and the torso still.

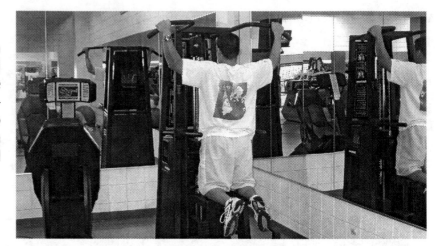

■ **4-5b. Bilateral bent-over row with dumbbells:**

Stand in a hip hinge position, with the knees soft, the abdominals contracted, and the spine held in its ideal (neutral) alignment, and with the neck in line with the spine. Perform a bilateral row in the low-row position, with the upper arms brushing the sides, while engaging the lats. Maintain a stable torso at all times.

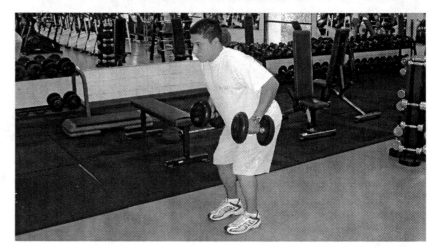

LEVEL 6: Add Balance, Increased Function, Speed, and/or Rotation

■ **4-6a. Standing unilateral low row balance:**

Placing one foot on a half-foam roller, balance with the abdominals contracted and the pelvis, spine, and neck in neutral. Place the non-working hand on the same-side thigh for support. Facing the low pulley, grasp the handle and perform a row in the low-row position, with the upper arm brushing the ribcage. Keep the shoulders level and the torso stable throughout.

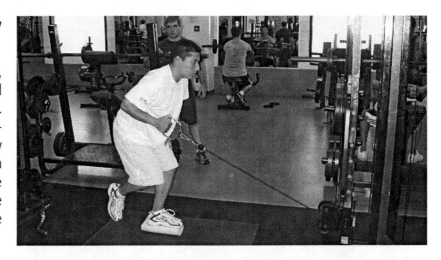

■ **4-6b. Low-row squat/lunge with tubing:**

With a partner anchoring the tubing, start by performing a one-leg squat, with the right knee extended in front. Return to the starting position through a crane (stork/bent knee) balance position and perform a back lunge with the right leg. Repeat 8-12 times with the right leg, simultaneously performing a bilateral low row with the tubing. Keep the pelvis, spine, neck, and wrists neutral, and the abdominals contracted. Maintain a stable, upright torso throughout.

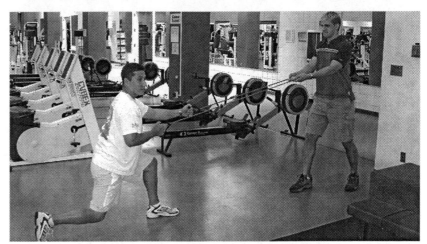

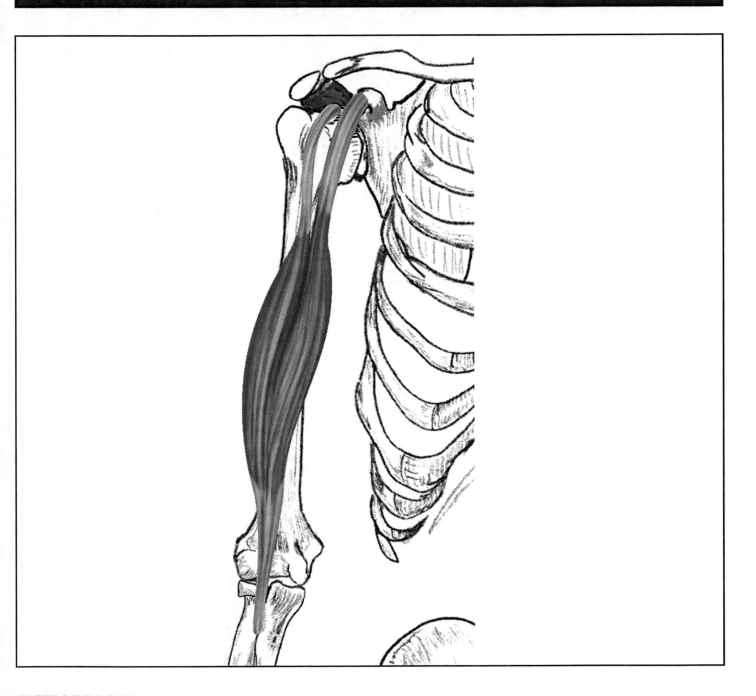

BICEPS BRACHII

Primary Joint Action:

- Elbow flexion

Assists with supination and shoulder flexion.

LEVEL 1: Isolate/Educate

■ **5-1a. Seated unilateral elbow flexion:**

Sit on a bench with the spine, neck, and scapulae in neutral, holding the upper arms close to the ribs. Exhale, keep the wrist straight, and flex one elbow at a time, engaging the biceps.

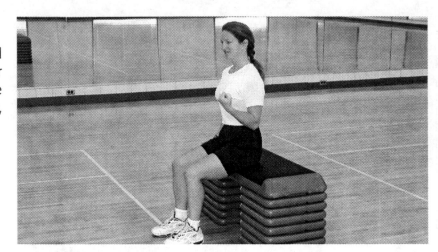

■ **5-1b. Seated bilateral elbow flexion:**

Sit on a bench with the spine, neck, and scapulae in neutral, holding the upper arms close to the ribs. Exhale, keep the wrists straight and flex both elbows, engaging the biceps.

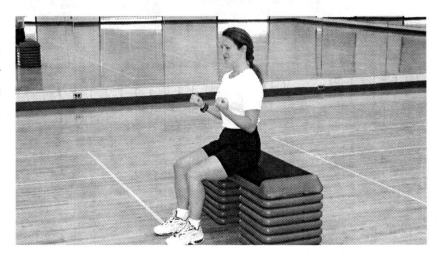

LEVEL 2: Isolate/Educate with Resistance

5-2a. Paramount biceps VR machine:

Sit at the machine with the spine, neck, and scapulae in neutral. Adjust the pads so that the cam is even with the elbow joints. Keeping the wrists straight, slowly flex the elbows, contracting the biceps.

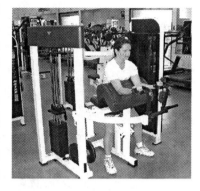

5-2b. Seated bilateral curls with dumbbells:

Sit on a bench with the spine, neck, and scapulae in neutral, holding the upper arms close to the ribs. Exhale, keep the wrists straight, and flex both elbows, engaging the biceps.

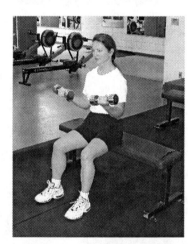

5-2c. Bilateral curls prone on an incline bench:

Lie prone on a bench, with the torso stabilized and the arms hanging straight down. Grasping the dumbbells in both hands, slowly flex the elbows, contracting the biceps and keeping the wrists in neutral.

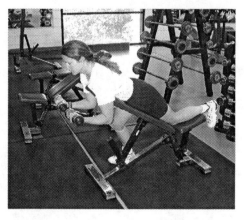

5-2d. Bilateral curl supine on an incline bench:

Lie supine on a bench with the torso stabilized, the abdominals engaged, and the arms hanging straight down. Slowly flex the elbows, keeping the wrists straight, while contracting the biceps.

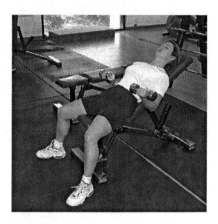

5-2e. Concentration curls:

Sit on the end of the bench and hinge the hips so that the spine is kept in a neutral alignment. Maintain the neck, scapulae, and wrists in neutral. Place the non-working hand on the opposite thigh for support and allow the working-side elbow to be braced against the inside of the thigh. Smoothly curl the weight, consciously contracting the biceps.

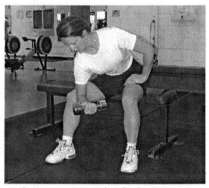

LEVEL 3: Add Functional Training Positions

■ **5-3a. Standing bilateral curl at the wall:**

Stand against a wall, with the knees soft, and the pelvis, spine, neck, and scapulae in neutral. Holding the elbows against the sides, curl the bar slowly upwards. Maintain the wrists in neutral.

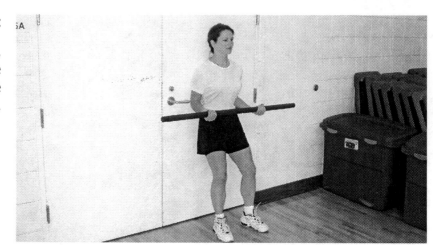

■ **5-3b. Standing alternating unilateral curls:**

Stand with the knees soft, and the pelvis, spine, neck, and scapulae in neutral alignment. Keep the arms down, with the palms facing in. Keeping the shoulders level and the upper arms pressed to the ribs, slowly flex the right elbow, simultaneously performing radio-ulnar supination (turning the palm to face up). Keep the wrists neutral. Repeat on the other side.

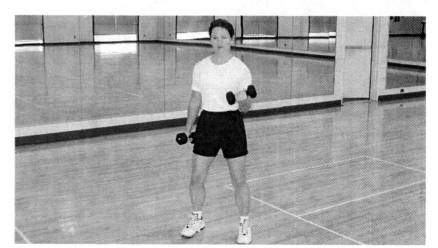

■ **5-3c. Standing bilateral curls with tubing:**

Stand on tubing, with the knees soft, and the pelvis, spine, neck, and scapulae in neutral. Grasp the handles in both hands and, keeping the wrists straight, slowly flex both elbows, engaging the biceps.

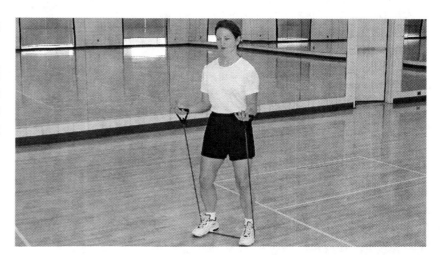

LEVEL 4: Combine Increased Function with Resistance

■ **5-4a. Standing bilateral curl at low pulley:**

Using an EZ curl bar, stand facing the low pulley in good alignment. Keep the knees soft, and the pelvis, spine, neck, and scapulae in neutral. Holding the upper arms close to the ribs and maintaining neutral wrists, slowly curl the bar upwards, exhaling.

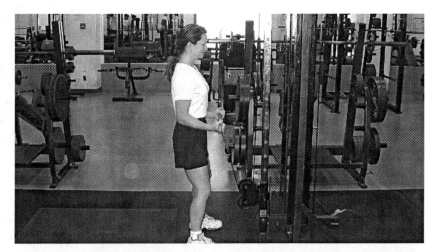

■ **5-4b. Standing unilateral curl at a low pulley:**

Facing away from the low pulley, stagger the feet so that a straight line exists from the back heel to the head. Keep the knees soft, the abdominals contracted, and the spine, neck, and scapulae in neutral. Place the non-working hand on the thigh for stability. Grasp the handle in the working hand and slowly flex the elbow, maintaining a neutral wrist.

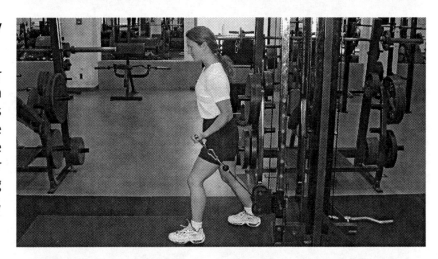

■ **5-4c. Preacher curl on a stability ball:**

Lie prone over a stability ball with the ball under the chest and the upper arms supported. Maintain a straight line from the heels to the head. The feet may be brought together to increase the balance challenge. Grasping the weights with both hands and keeping the wrists straight, slowly flex both elbows, engaging the biceps.

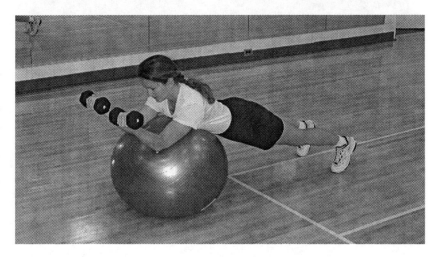

LEVEL 5: Multi-Muscle Groups with Increased Resistance and Core Challenge

■ **5-5a. Biceps curls with front lunges:**

Perform alternating front lunges, with the torso erect, and the pelvis, spine, neck, and scapulae in neutral. Maintain proper front-knee alignment, with the knee flexed no greater than 90°; keep the abdominals contracted. Simultaneously flex both elbows during the descent phase, engaging the biceps.

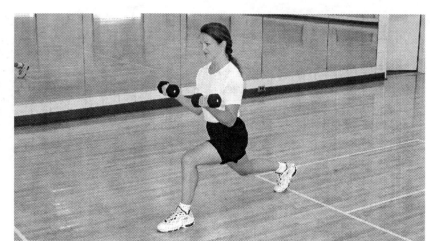

■ **5-5b. One-arm curl, one-arm kickback, stationary lunge:**

Perform a stationary lunge, with the torso erect, and the pelvis, spine, neck, and scapulae in neutral. Maintain proper front-knee alignment, with the knee flexed no greater than 90°; keep the abdominals contracted. Simultaneously perform a bicep curl with one arm, while executing a triceps kickback with the other. Keep both wrists straight and hold the upper arm on the triceps-side, parallel to the floor.

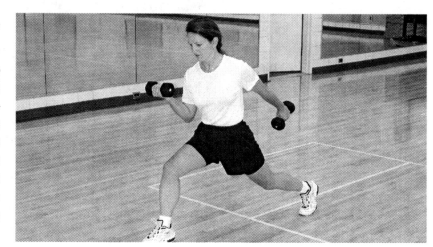

LEVEL 6: Add Balance, Increased Function, Speed, and/or Rotation

■ **5-6a. 4-count balance:**

While balancing on one foot with the knee soft and the pelvis, spine, neck, and scapulae in neutral, perform the following 4-count move: 1) flex the shoulders, 2) flex the elbows, 3) extend the elbows, and 4) bring the shoulders back to neutral. Keep the wrists straight and engage the biceps and anterior deltoids.

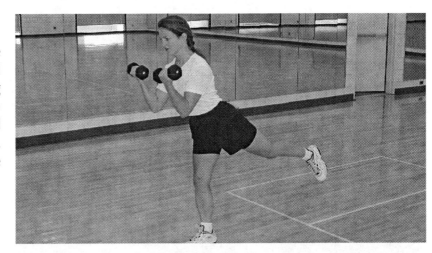

■ **5-6b. Preacher curl on a stability ball with balance:**

Lie prone over a stability ball with the ball under the chest and the upper arms supported. Maintaining a straight line from the heels to the head, lift one foot and balance, challenging the core muscles. Grasping the weights with both hands and keeping the wrists straight, slowly flex both elbows, engaging the biceps.

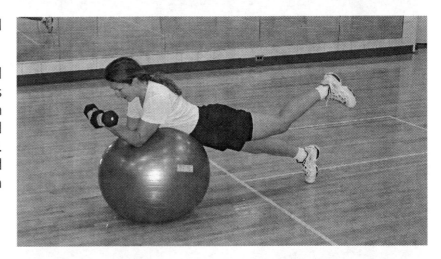

■ **5-6c. Standing unilateral curl at a low pulley with balance:**

Standing at the low pulley, place one foot on a half foam roller and balance, keeping the knees soft, the abdominals contracted, and the spine, neck, and scapulae in neutral. The non-working hand may be placed on the thigh for stability. Contracting the abdominals, grasp the handle in the working hand and slowly flex the elbow, engaging the bicep.

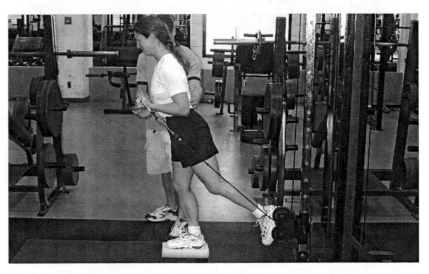

CHAPTER SIX
Triceps

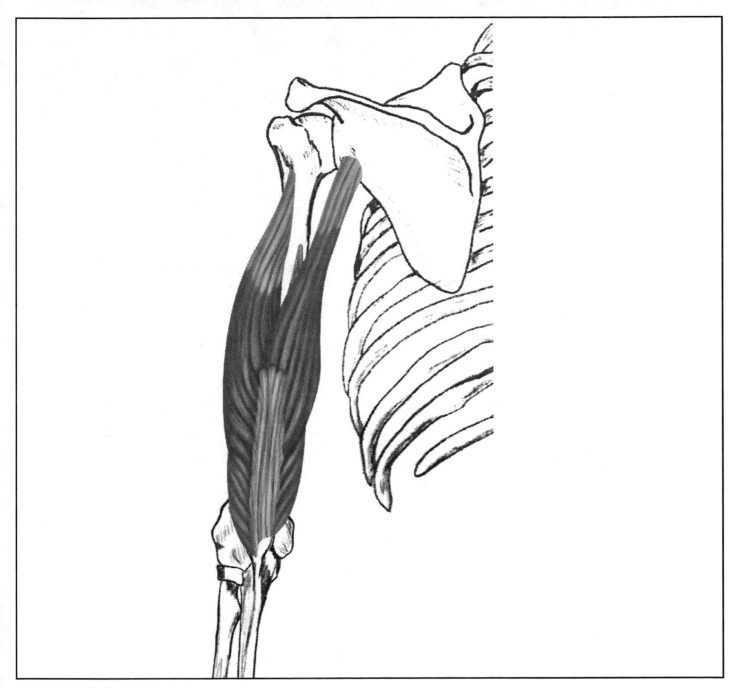

TRICEPS BRACHII

Primary Joint Action:

• Elbow extension

Assists with shoulder extension and shoulder adduction.

LEVEL 1: Isolate/Educate

■ **6-1a. Supine unilateral elbow extension:**

Lie in a supine position with the knees bent, and the spine and neck in neutral. Start with the working arm vertical/perpendicular to the floor. Flex the elbow and slowly return to vertical, engaging the triceps.

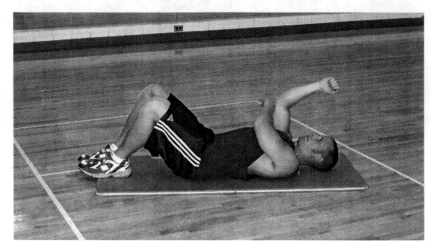

■ **6-1b. Supine bilateral elbow extension:**

Lie supine with the knees bent, and the spine and neck in neutral. Start with both arms vertical/perpendicular to the floor. Flex the elbows and slowly return to vertical, engaging the triceps.

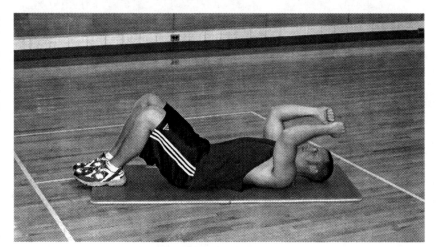

LEVEL 2: Isolate/Educate with Resistance

■ 6-2a. Supine bilateral extension with partner resistance:

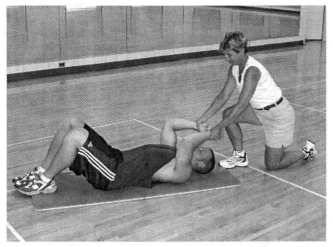

Lie in a supine position with the knees bent, and the spine and neck in neutral. Start with the working arms vertical/perpendicular to the floor. Flex the elbows and slowly return to vertical, engaging the triceps, while the partner applies manual resistance against the forearms. Keep the upper arms still.

■ 6-2b. Supine bilateral extension with a dumbbell (skullcrusher):

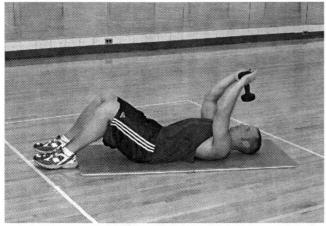

Lie in a supine position with the knees bent, and the spine and neck in neutral. Start with both arms vertical/perpendicular to the floor. Hold the end of one dumbbell with both hands. Carefully flex the elbows and slowly return to vertical, engaging the triceps and keeping the upper arms stable.

■ 6-2c. Bilateral elbow extension on a Cybex VR machine:

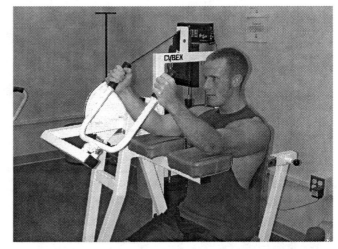

Sit with the shoulders flexed, the scapulae depressed, and the elbows flexed on a pad, while grasping the handles. Slowly extend the elbows, engaging the triceps. Maintain spinal stability throughout.

■ 6-2d. Badger pressdown VR machine:

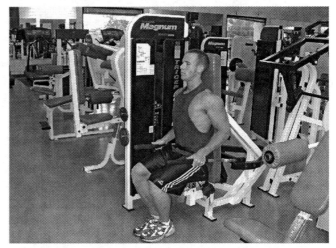

Sit with the spine and the neck in neutral. Slowly press the handles down, extending the elbows and consciously contracting the triceps.

LEVEL 3: Add Functional Training Positions

■ **6-3a. Kneeling unilateral elbow extension (kickback):**

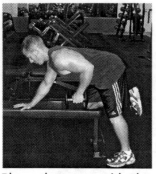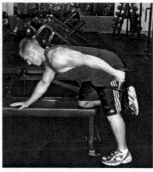

Place the same-side hand and knee on a bench. Hinge at the hips; keep the spine, neck, and scapulae in neutral, and the shoulders level. Place the working arm parallel to the floor and, using a dumbbell, slowly extend the elbow, engaging the triceps. Keep the wrist straight.

■ **6-3b. Standing unilateral pressdown with an elastic band/tube:**

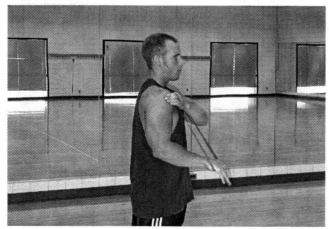

Stand in good alignment, with the knees soft, and the pelvis, spine, neck, and scapulae in neutral. Anchoring a band/tube to the right shoulder, hold the end of the band/tube in the right hand. Extend the right elbow, engaging the triceps. Adjust the tension of the band/tube to achieve fatigue within 10-15 repetitions. Repeat on the other side.

■ **6-3c. Standing unilateral overhead extension (French press) with a tube:**

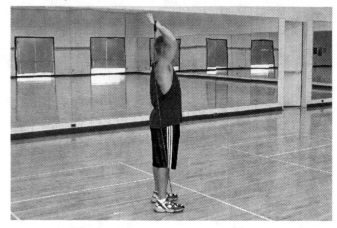

Stand with the right foot on the end of the tube, and hold the opposite end of the tube in the right hand behind the head. Stand in good alignment, with the knees soft, and the pelvis, spine, neck, and scapulae in neutral. The right elbow points directly up. Extend the right elbow overhead, keeping the upper arm stationary.

■ **6-3d. Standing unilateral triceps extension (kickback) with partner:**

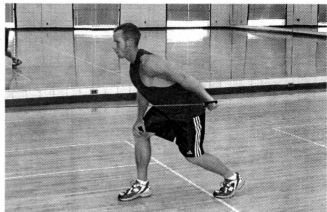

Have the partner hold one end of the tube at approximately waist height. Stand with the feet staggered, with the non-working hand on the same-side thigh. Keep the spine, neck, and scapulae in neutral, and the upper arm of the working-side parallel to the floor. Extend the elbow back, contracting the triceps. Keep the rest of the body stable.

LEVEL 4: Combine Increased Function with Resistance

■ 6-4a. Standing pressdown at a high pulley:

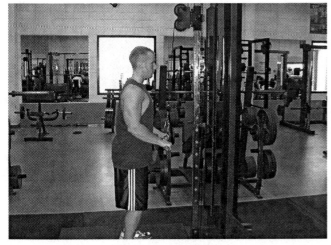

Stand in good alignment, with the knees soft, and the spine, neck, pelvis, and scapulae in neutral. Keep the upper arms close to the ribs. Slowly press the bar down, and then release upwards, keeping the upper arms still. Repeat.

■ 6-4b. Bent-over bilateral elbow extension (kickbacks):

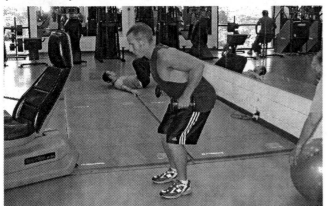

Partially squat with the weight over the heels, the knees behind the toes, the tailbone pointing back, and the spine, neck, and scapulae in neutral. Hold completely stable, with the abdominals contracted, while performing bilateral kickbacks with weights. The elbows are the only moving joints; keep the shoulders level and still.

■ 6-4c. Unilateral elbow extension on a Free Motion VR machine:

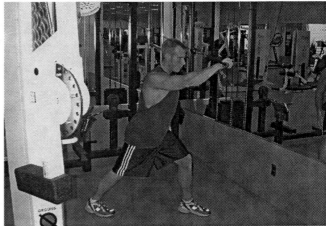

Stand facing away from the high-pulley unit. Stagger the feet and maintain a straight line from the back heel through the head; keep the spine, pelvis, neck, and scapulae in neutral. Start with the working arm flexed, the hand grasping the handle, and the upper arm parallel to the floor. Smoothly extend the elbow, engaging the triceps and keeping the wrist straight.

■ 6-4d. Bilateral elbow extension (kickbacks) with a partner:

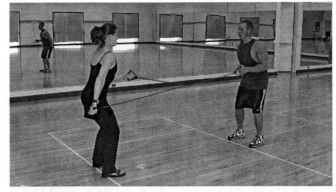

Interlock the tubes and step away from each other to an appropriate distance for optimal resistance. Both partners perform a partial squat, with weight over the heels, knees behind the toes, tailbones pointing back, and spines, necks, and scapulae in neutral. Both individuals hold completely stable, with abdominals contracted, while performing bilateral kickbacks. The elbows are the only moving joints.

LEVEL 5: Multi-Muscle Groups with Increased Resistance and Core Challenge

■ **6-5a. Stairmaster Gravitron dips:**

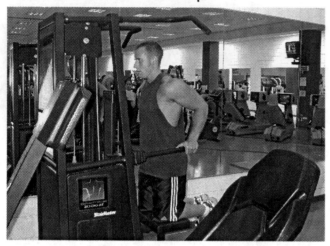

Using the assisted resistance device, kneel on the pad with hands on the bars, and shoulders away from the ears, with the elbows straight, but not hyperextended. Slowly lower the body, with the elbows directly behind the body, while keeping the scapulae depressed, and the spine, pelvis, and neck in neutral. Extend the elbows, lifting the body upwards. Gradually decrease the amount of weight assisting the dips.

■ **6-5b. Triceps push-up:**

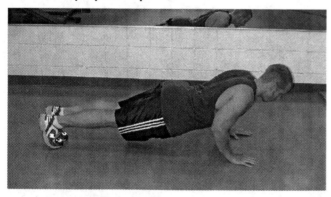

Can be performed on either the knees or the toes. Place the hands under the shoulders and hold the spine, pelvis, neck, and scapulae in neutral. Slowly flex the elbows, lowering the body; keep the upper arms against the ribcage. Avoid flaring the elbows away from the body. Return to the starting position, engaging the triceps.

■ **6-5c. Dips off a bench:**

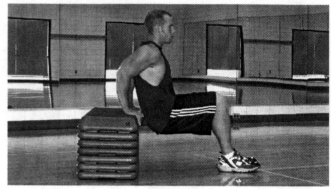

Place the hands on a bench, directly in line with the shoulders. Start with the knees bent and progress to a knees-straight position to increase the level of difficulty. Slowly flex the elbows directly behind the body (avoid flaring) and then extend, contracting the triceps. Keep the scapulae depressed and the neck in neutral.

■ **6-5d. Alternating front lunge with a bilateral triceps kickback:**

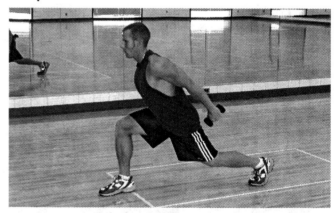

Step forward with one foot into a front lunge, while simultaneously performing bilateral kickbacks. Return to a standing position; keep the upper arms parallel to the floor. While lunging, keep the torso completely upright, and the pelvis, spine, neck, and scapulae in neutral. Alternate legs.

LEVEL 6: Add Balance, Increased Function, Speed, and/or Rotation

6-6a. Dips off a stability ball:

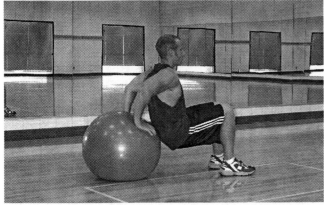

Place both hands on the stability ball and balance with the hips off the ball, and the feet on the floor. The level of difficulty may be increased by progressing to a knees-straight position. Slowly flex the elbows, keeping the scapulae depressed and the neck in neutral. Extend, maintaining core stability and engaging the triceps.

6-6b. Unilateral elbow extension at mid-pulley with balance:

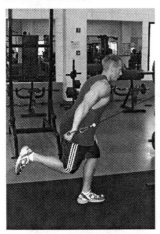
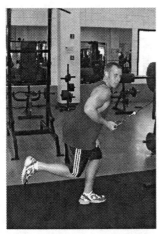

Stand balanced on one foot, with the same side hand on the thigh. Maintain a hip-hinge position, with the abdominals contracted and the spine, neck, and scapulae in neutral. Set the mid-pulley at approximately elbow height. Holding the handle with the working-side hand, extend the elbow back, engaging the triceps. Keep the shoulders level.

6-6c. Overhead medicine ball toss to a partner:

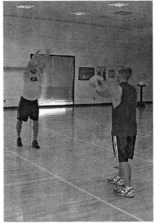
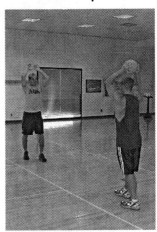

Stand in good alignment, with the knees soft, and the pelvis, spine, and neck in neutral. Hold the medicine ball behind the head in a French-press position, with the elbows pointing straight up. Extend the elbows and toss the ball to the partner, who utilizes the same position, while returning the ball.

6-6d. Overhead medicine ball toss to a partner with balance:

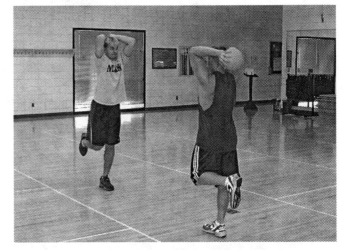

Balancing on one foot, stand in good alignment, with the knee soft, and the pelvis, spine, and neck in neutral. Hold the medicine ball behind the head in a French-press position, with the elbows pointing straight up. Extend the elbows and toss the ball to the partner, who utilizes the same position while returning the ball. Maintain balance on one foot throughout.

PART TWO: CORE PROGRESSIONS

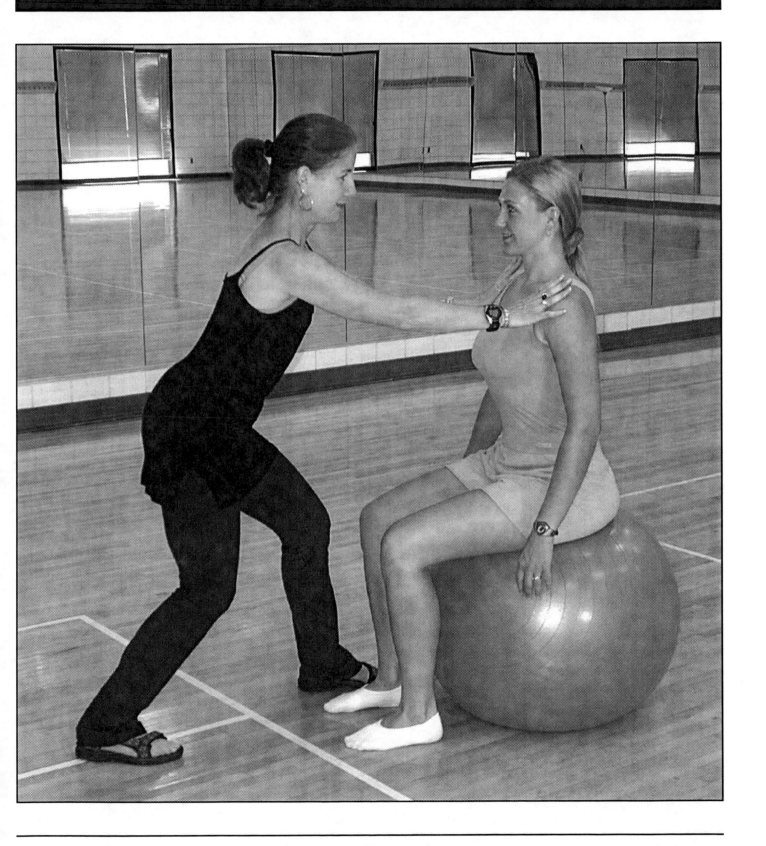

CHAPTER SEVEN
Abdominals as Prime Movers

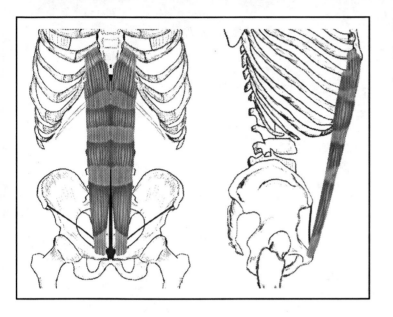

RECTUS ABDOMINIS

Primary Joint Action:

- Spinal flexion

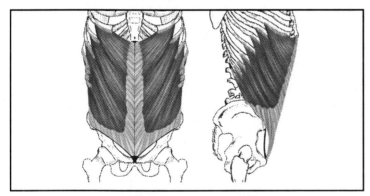

EXTERNAL OBLIQUES

EXTERNAL AND INTERNAL OBLIQUES

Primary Joint Actions:

- Spinal flexion
- Spinal rotation
- Spinal lateral flexion

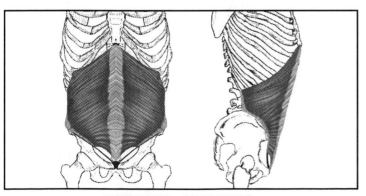

INTERNAL OBLIQUES

Note: The prime mover in all of the exercises in this chapter is either the rectus abdominis, the obliques, or both. The exercises may engage the transverse abdominis by vigorously exhaling on the crunch phase of each exercise and by compressing the abdominal wall inwards.

LEVEL 1: Isolate/Educate

■ **7-1a. Basic crunch:**

Lie with the feet up on the bench to minimize stress to the low back. Curl up approximately 30-40°, keeping the head and neck in line with the spine.

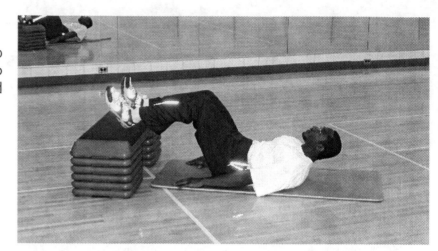

■ **7-1b. Basic oblique crunch:**

Lie with the feet up on the bench to minimize stress to the low back. Curl up approximately 30-40°, moving diagonally, with the ribs towards the opposite hip. Keep the hips and legs still and the head and neck in line with the spine.

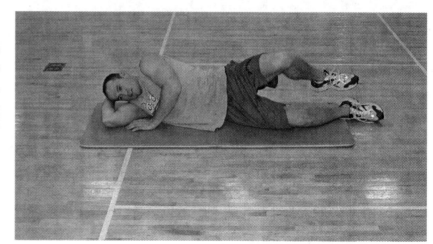

LEVEL 2: Isolate/Educate with Resistance

■ **7-2a. Basic crunch with the feet on the floor, and the hands behind the ears/head:**

Lie with the feet on the floor and the knees bent. Placing the hands behind the ears or the head increases the lever length, thus increasing the difficulty of the exercise slightly. Curl up approximately 30-40°, keeping the head and neck in line with the spine. Maintain a fist-sized space between the chin and the chest.

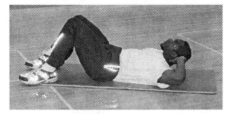

■ **7-2b. Basic oblique crunch with the feet on the floor, and the hands behind the ears/head:**

Lie with the feet on floor and the knees bent. Curl up approximately 30-40°, keeping the head and neck in line with the spine and moving diagonally. Stabilize the hips and legs; keep the elbows just barely visible in the peripheral vision.

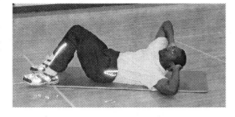

■ **7-2c. Ultimate crunch:**

Lie with the feet in the air, with the hands behind the ears or head. Curl both ends of the spine up together, lifting the ribs and pubic bone towards each other. Keep the head and neck in line with the spine, and avoid swinging the legs. Maintain the angle of hip flexion isometrically, while performing spinal flexion to challenge the rectus abdominis.

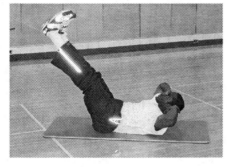

■ **7-2d. Quantum machine crunch:**

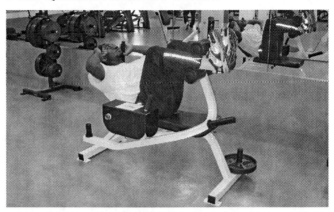

Keep the head and neck relaxed. Perform spinal flexion, while hollowing the abdominal wall inwards.

■ **7-2e. Nautilus curl machine:**

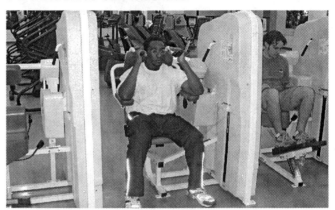

Adjust the machine so that hip flexion is minimized and the abdominal muscles are recruited through active spinal flexion. Exhale and pull the abdominal wall in while performing the movement.

LEVEL 3: Add Functional Training Positions

Note: This level is not included in this progression because it is very difficult to challenge the abdominals simply by moving to a standing or seated (i.e., a more functional) position. Resistance of some type must be added for sufficient overload, and this step occurs in Level #4 of this progression. However, the standing position without resistance is a possible option for pregnant women past their first trimester who are advised against exercising in the supine position.

LEVEL 3: Add Functional Training Positions

LEVEL 4: Combine Increased Function with Resistance

■ **7-4a. Kneeling crunch from a high pulley:**

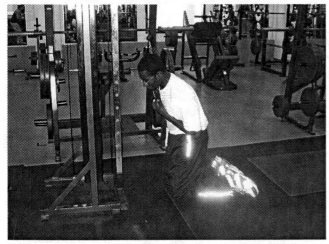

Hold ropes or a strap on either side of the neck. Kneel and stabilize the hips, legs, and pelvis. Perform spinal flexion, drawing the ribs towards the pelvis. Engage the abdominal wall, while exhaling.

■ **7-4b. Low pulley, knees over stability ball, ultimate crunch:**

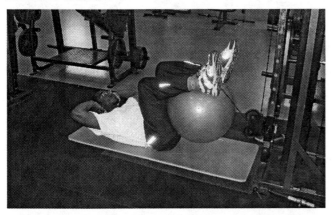

Place each ankle in a cuff attached to the low pulley. Lift the feet up and place over a stability ball. Using the knee flexors, hug the ball to the thighs with the feet. Contracting the abdominals, lift the pelvis towards the ribs. If desired, simultaneously flex the ribs towards the pelvis.

■ **7-4c. Standing crunch with Free Motion equipment:**

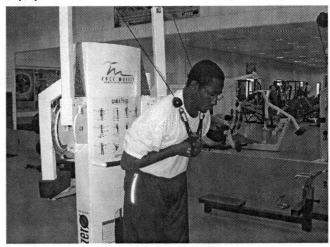

Stand facing away from the machine and stabilize the entire lower body, keeping the knees soft. Squeeze the buttocks to help prevent hip flexion. Exhaling, pull the abdominal wall in and perform spinal flexion, keeping the head and neck in line with the spine.

■ **7-4d. Standing oblique crunch with Free Motion equipment:**

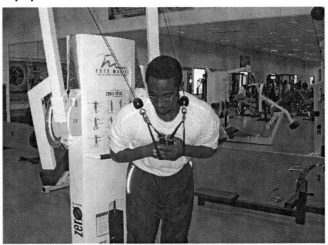

Stand facing away from the machine and stabilize the entire lower body, keeping the knees soft. Squeeze the buttocks to help prevent hip flexion. Exhaling, pull the abdominal wall in and perform a diagonal movement with the upper torso, keeping the head and neck in line with the spine.

LEVEL 5: Multi-Muscle Groups with Increased Resistance and Core Challenge

■ **7-5a. Bicycle:**

Curl the upper torso into 30°-40° of spinal flexion, keeping the head and neck in line with the spine. Maintaining this position and moving slowly with control, flex— alternating the hips and knees, while rotating the upper spine. Stabilize the pelvis and lower back on the floor.

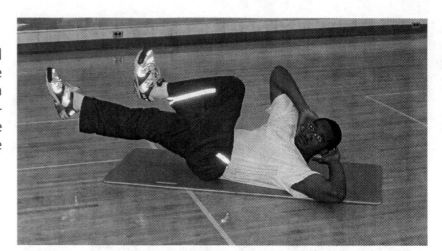

■ **7-5b. Unilateral hip flexion with arm reach:**

Bring one leg up, while keeping the opposite foot on the floor, with the knee bent. Simultaneously reach both arms up to touch the shin, ankle, or foot, while flexing the spine 30°-40°. Maintain pelvic and lower-back stability and avoid rocking side to side or using momentum.

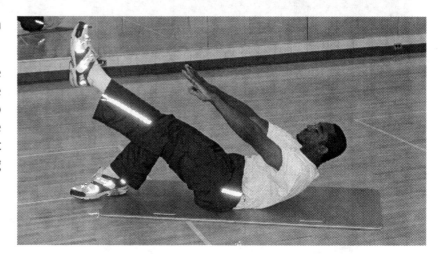

LEVEL 6: Add Balance, Increased Function, Speed, and/or Rotation

■ 7-6a. Stability ball crunch:

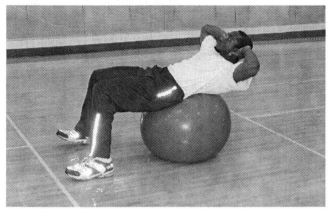

This exercise can be performed in a variety of positions: inclined (easier), parallel to the floor (as shown), or declined (harder). The level of difficulty of the exercise may also be increased by bringing the feet closer together. Avoid extending the back too far over the ball if back problems exist. Support the head with the hands behind the head, taking care to keep the neck in line with the spine and a fist-sized distance between the chin and the chest.

■ 7-6b. Stability ball oblique crunch:

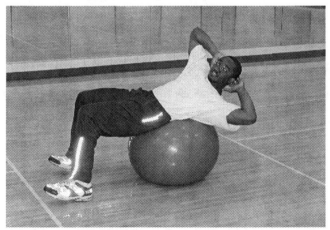

Avoid extending the back too far over the ball if back problems exist. Support the head with the hands behind the head, keeping the neck in line with the spine and a fist-sized distance between the chin and the chest. Move the ribs towards the opposite hip.

■ 7-6c. Roman chair:

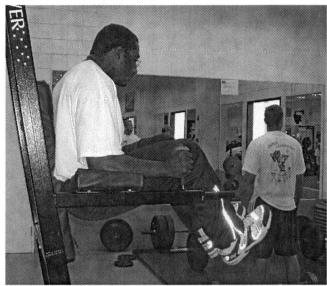

Isometrically, hold the knees and hips at an angle that is approximately 90° of flexion. The joint action necessary to actively train the abdominal muscles is spinal flexion. Contract the abdominals and pull the pubic bone upwards towards the ribcage without swinging or dynamically moving the legs.

■ 7-6d. Stability ball crunch on one foot:

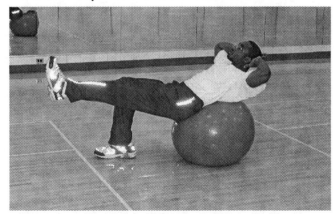

This exercise is the same as was detailed for exercises 7-6a and 7-6b, except that it is made considerably more difficult when performed with one foot lifted. Stabilize the hips and lower spine on the ball. Support the head and neck with the hands, keeping a fist-sized distance between the chin and the chest.

CHAPTER EIGHT

Erector Spinae as a Prime Mover

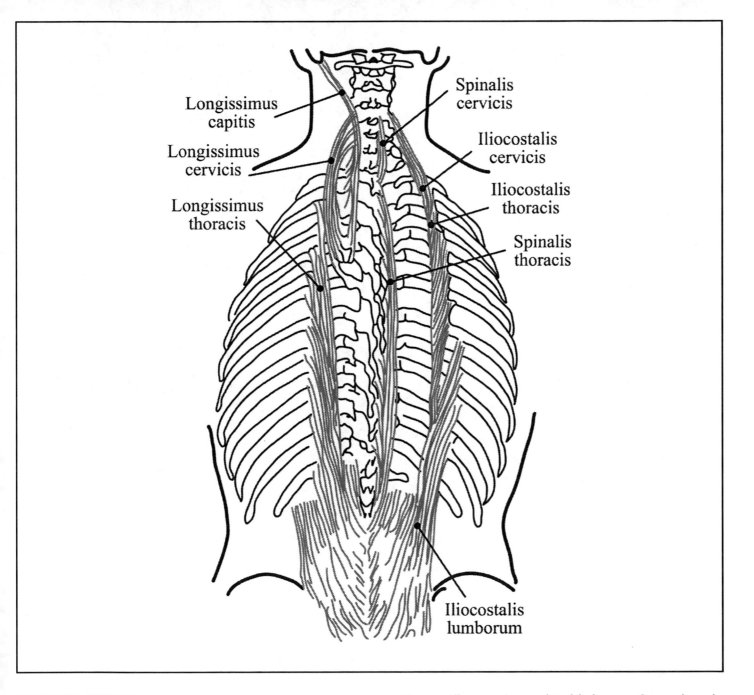

Longissimus capitis

Longissimus cervicis

Longissimus thoracis

Spinalis cervicis

Iliocostalis cervicis

Iliocostalis thoracis

Spinalis thoracis

Iliocostalis lumborum

ERECTOR SPINAE

Primary Joint Action:

- Spinal extension

- Note: All exercises should be performed only through a pain free range of motion, while moving slowly without momentum. Some controversy exists regarding whether to do exercises that involve extreme hyperextension, especially if the exercise utilizes additional resistance.

LEVEL 1: Isolate/Educate

■ **8-1a. Prone extension, with the hands at the sides:**

Lie in a prone position, with the neck in line with the spine, and the chin slightly tucked. Contract the abdominals and tighten the buttocks. Keeping the hips and the lowest ribs on the mat, lift the upper torso, while maintaining proper neck alignment.

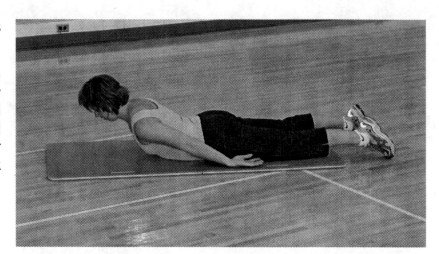

■ **8-1b. Prone extension, modified cobra exercise:**

Lie in a prone position, with the neck in line with the spine, the chin slightly tucked, and the hands on the floor near the shoulders. Engaging the lower back muscles, lift the upper torso, while simultaneously sliding the elbows into a propped position under the shoulders. Under control, slowly lower back to the starting position. Unlike the modified held cobra stretch, this option is a strengthening exercise. Perform 8-12 repetitions.

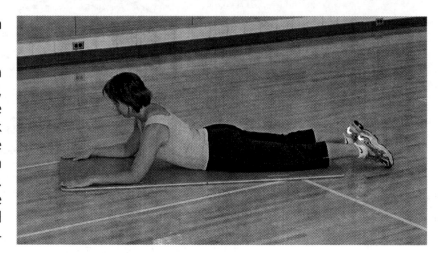

LEVEL 2: Isolate/Educate with Resistance

■ **8-2a. Prone position, hands out to the side in a "goalpost" position:**

Lie in a prone position, with the neck in line with the spine, and the chin slightly tucked. Contract the abdominals and tighten the buttocks. Keeping the hips and the lowest ribs on the mat, lift the upper torso, while maintaining the neck in proper alignment. Placing the hands in a "goalpost" position increases the lever length and the level of the resistance involved in performing the exercise against gravity.

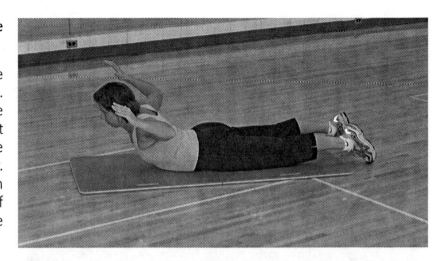

■ **8-2b. Prone extension using the opposite arm and leg:**

Lie in a prone position, with the neck in line with the spine, and the chin slightly tucked. Maintaining the stability of the middle torso, smoothly lift the opposite arm and leg. The head lifts and lowers naturally in line with the spine. Alternate sides.

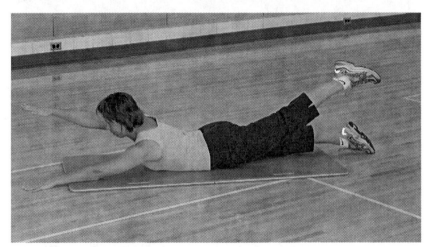

LEVEL 3: Add Functional Training Positions

Note: This level is not included in this progression because it is very difficult to challenge the erector spinae muscles simply by moving to a standing or seated (i.e., more functional) position. Resistance of some type must be added for sufficient overload. This step occurs in level #4 of this exercise progression.

LEVEL 3: Add Functional Training Positions

LEVEL 4: Combine Increased Function with Resistance

■ **8-4a. Nautilus seated back extension VR machine:**

This exercise can be performed in two ways. First, start with the spine flexed forward and the abdominals contracted. Extend backwards into a neutral sitting position. Repeat. Second, start with the spine flexed forward and the abdominals contracted. Extend the spine backwards through it's full, comfortable range of motion, past neutral into hyperextension, stopping if any discomfort occurs. This machine has a range-limiter device if low back pain creates any discomfort while exercising through the full range of motion.

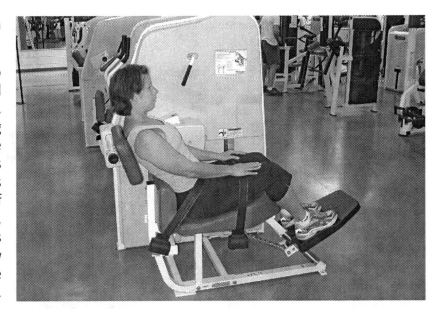

■ **8-4b. 45-degree extension chair:**

Flex the spine at a 45° angle and extend the torso, using the low-back muscles, assisted by the hamstrings. Hyperextend slightly (10-15°) in order to be able to "look up at airplanes" in the future!

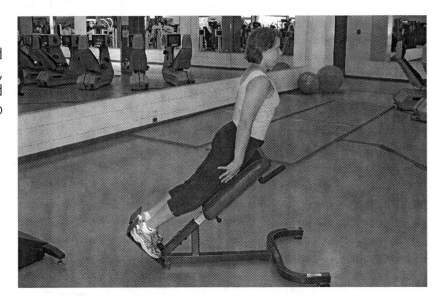

LEVEL 5: Multi-Muscle Groups with Increased Resistance and Core Challenge

■ **8-5a. Prone extension combined with reverse pec-dec:**

Perform spinal extension as previously described, while simultaneously retracting the scapulae and engaging the mid-trapezius and rhomboid muscles.

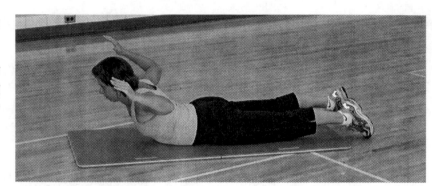

■ **8-5b. Pilates "double heel kick":**

Lie in a prone position with the toes pointed, the legs extended straight, the chin down, and the hands clasped behind the back. Kick both heels twice towards the buttocks, flexing the knees. Then, extend the straight legs up and out, while extending the spine and retracting the scapulae, pulling the arms back and up. Keep the head in line with the spine.

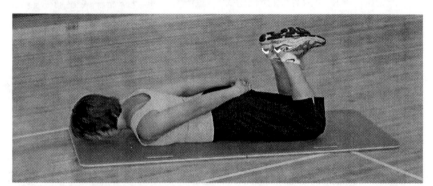

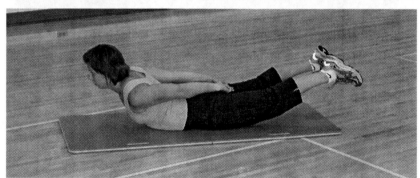

■ **8-5c. Pilates swimming:**

Lie in a prone position with the toes pointed, the legs extended straight, the chin down, and the arms reaching overhead. Lift the upper and lower body together, keeping the spine in extension and the neck in neutral. Flutter the arms and legs. Keep the pelvis and the lower ribs in contact with the floor, maintaining a stable torso.

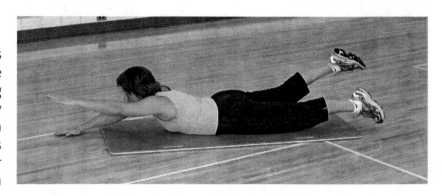

LEVEL 6: Add Balance, Increased Function, Speed, and/or Rotation

■ **8-6a. Stability ball extension, with the arms at the sides:**

Lie in a prone position with the ball under the abdominals. Moving the feet far apart enhances stability; bringing the feet together decreases stability, thus increasing the balance challenge. Keeping the neck in neutral, extend the spine. Increase the level of difficulty of the exercise by bringing the hands either to the ears or overhead for longer lever length.

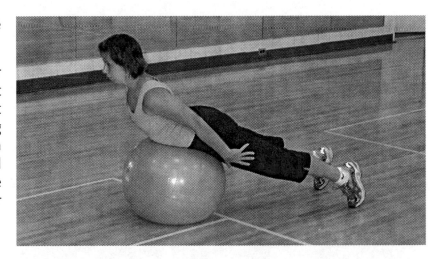

■ **8-6b. Stability ball extension, with one foot on the floor:**

While extending the spine, lift one foot off the floor. Alternate with each repetition, keeping the lower torso stable.

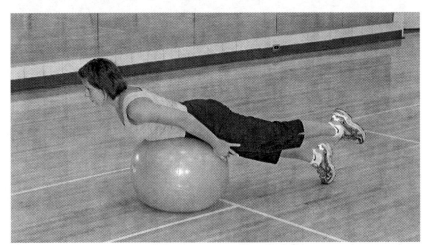

CHAPTER NINE

Torso Muscles as Stabilizers

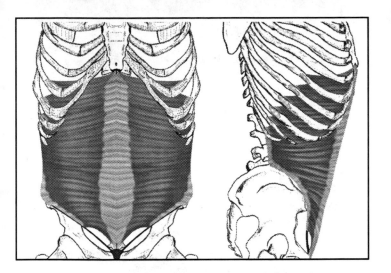

TRANSVERSE ABDOMINIS

Primary Joint Actions:

- Abdominal compression
- Vigorous exhalation and expulsion

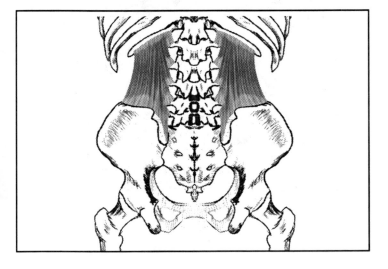

QUADRATUS LUMBORUM

Primary Joint Action:

- Spinal lateral flexion

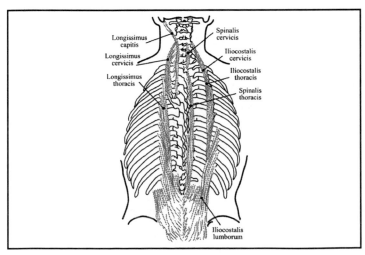

ERECTOR SPINAE

Primary Joint Action:

- Spinal extension

Muscles challenged include: rectus abdominis, obliques, transverse abdominis, quatratus lumborum, erector spinae, and multifidus. In this progression, the goal is to isometrically challenge the core muscles to keep the spine in neutral no matter how the overload is applied. In a neutral spine, all four curves exist and are maintained in their ideal alignment to each other. Scapular stability is important too. Stabilizing muscles for the scapula include the trapezius, rhomboids, levator scapulae, serratus anterior, and pectoralis minor. A neutral shoulder girdle is depressed (not elevated), in a position midway between protraction and retraction.

LEVEL 1: Isolate/Educate

■ **9-1a. Supine unilateral heel slide:**

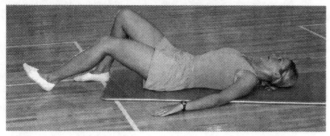

Lie in a supine position with both knees bent, the feet on the floor, the spine in neutral, and the abdominals hollowed. With control, slowly slide one heel along the floor until the knee is straight, then return. Alternate sides, keeping the pelvis, spine, scapulae, and neck perfectly still. Maintain abdominal hollowing throughout.

■ **9-1b. Supine bridge:**

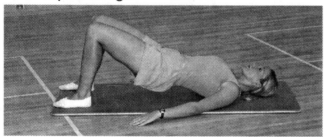

Lie in a supine position with both knees bent, the feet on the floor, the spine in neutral, and the abdominals hollowed. Keeping the spine completely still, press the feet into the floor and extend the hips. Pause, while maintaining the spine and pelvis in neutral, and then slowly lower.

■ **9-1c. All fours table top:**

On the hands and knees, place the spine, pelvis, scapulae, and neck in a neutral alignment. Engage the abdominals, lifting the belly upwards without moving the spine. Focus on finding and maintaining a true neutral, stable alignment.

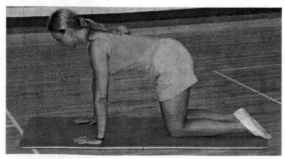

■ **9-1d. Prone opposite arm and leg hold:**

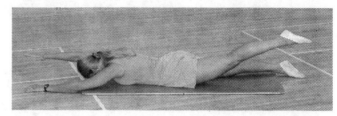

Lie in a prone position, with the toes pointed, the legs extended straight, the buttocks squeezed, the arms overhead, and the neck in alignment. Contract the abdominals and keep the hips and lower ribs in even contact with the floor. Slowly lift the opposite arm and leg. Pause, then lower and alternate sides, maintaining torso stability.

■ **9-1e. Side plank on the elbow and hip:**

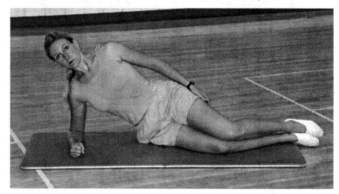

Lie on the side, up on the elbow. Lift the bottom ribs up away from the floor; keep the shoulders down, away from the neck and head. Place the spine, ribs, scapulae, and neck in neutral. Focus on maintaining stable alignment.

LEVEL 2: Isolate/Educate with Resistance

■ **9-2a. Knee fold:**

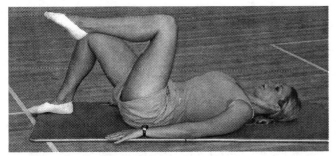

Lie in a supine position, with both knees bent, the feet on the floor, the spine in neutral, and the abdominals hollowed. With control, lift one knee and "fold" it in towards the torso, keeping the entire torso perfectly still. Lower the knee and touch the toes to the floor, maintaining the torso in neutral. Repeat. Increase the level of difficulty of performing the exercise by very slowly alternating the legs.

■ **9-2b. Dead bug:**

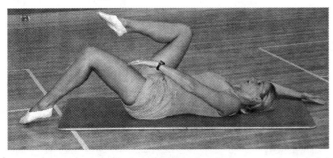

Start with the exercise described in 9-2a; then add arm movement, moving the same side-arm and leg. Increase the difficulty of the exercise by lengthening the arms, legs, or both. The goal is to keep the torso absolutely still, neutral, and stable throughout.

■ **9-2c. Bridge with balance:**

Lie in a supine position with both knees bent, the feet on the floor, the spine in neutral, and the abdominals hollowed. Keeping the spine completely still, press the feet into the floor and extend the hips. Pause, while maintaining the spine and pelvis in neutral. Then slowly lift one leg, keeping the pelvis and hips completely still.

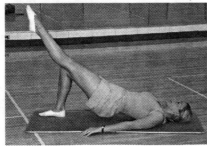

■ **9-2d. Quadruped:**

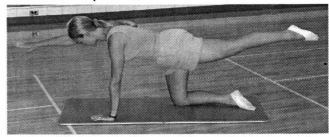

On the hands and knees, place the spine, pelvis, scapulae, and neck in a neutral alignment. Engage the abdominals, lifting the belly upwards without moving the spine. Extend one leg back and the opposite arm forward, while maintaining a neutral, stable alignment. Without shifting the spine, neck, or pelvis, switch to the other side.

■ **9-2e. Bent-elbow plank (hover):**

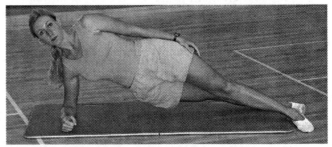

Maintain an ideal alignment while on the elbows and toes. Contract the abdominals, keeping the neck, scapulae, spine, and pelvis in neutral. Hold for 15-60 seconds.

■ **9-2f. Side plank on the elbow and feet:**

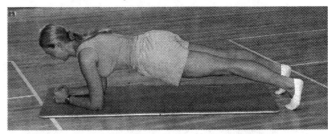

Support the body's weight on the elbow and feet. The feet may be scissored or stacked on top of each other. Square the torso to the front, pressing the scapulae into neutral and keeping the shoulders away from the ears. The spine and neck should be in a straight line. Contract the abdominals, keeping the neck, spine, and pelvis in neutral.

LEVEL 3: Add Functional Training Positions

■ **9-3a. Seated spinal twist:**

Sit on the floor, with the legs straight, the toes pointed, and the spine, neck, and scapulae in neutral. Use a pad under the edge of the buttocks if it is difficult to sit squarely on the sitting bones (ischial tuberosities). With the arms at shoulder height and the scapulae depressed, twist slowly to one side,

return to the starting position, and then twist to the other side. Repeat. The goal is to maintain a perfect sitting alignment throughout.

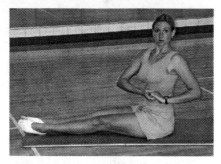

■ **9-3b. Plank:**

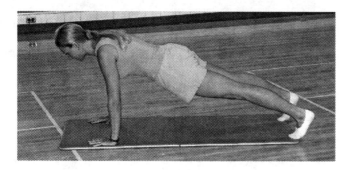

Maintain an ideal alignment while on the hands and toes. Contract the abdominals, keeping the neck, scapulae, spine and pelvis in neutral. Hold for 15-60 seconds.

■ **9-3c. Side Plank on the hand and foot:**

Support the body's weight on the hand and feet. The feet may be scissored or stacked on top of each other. Square the torso to the front, pressing the scapulae into neutral and keeping the shoulders

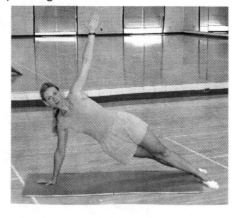

away from the ears. The spine and neck should be in a straight line. Contract the abdominals, keeping the neck, spine, and pelvis in neutral. Hold for 15-60 seconds.

■ **9-3d. Squat with arm scissors:**

Squat with the weight over the heels, the knees behind the toes, the tailbone pointing back, and the spine, neck, and scapulae in neutral. Hold completely stable, with the abdominals contracted, while slowly scissoring the arms back and forth.

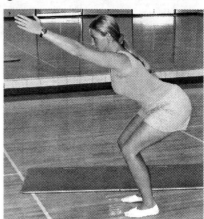

■ **9-3e. Standing hip hinge:**

Bending from the hips, keep the knees soft, the tailbone back, and the spine, neck, and scapulae in neutral. Avoid rounding the spine (hanging on long ligaments); contract the abdominals. Hold the position with the arms at sides, or, for more overload, with the arms overhead.

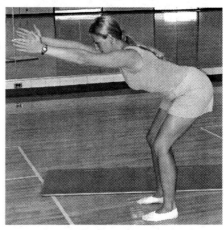

LEVEL 4: Combine Increased Function with Resistance

■ 9-4a. Seated resistance from a partner:

Sitting with an ideal alignment, have a partner apply pressure from the front; hold for 15-30 seconds. Repeat with the partner applying pressure from behind. The goal is to maintain a perfect sitting posture for ever-increasing periods of time.

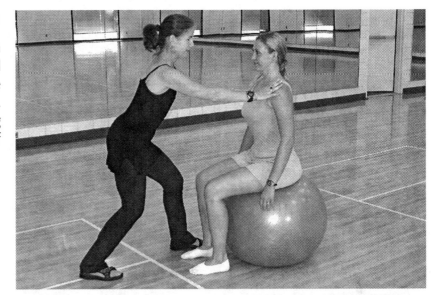

■ 9-4b. V-sit:

Start the exercise by sitting on the floor in an ideal alignment, with the knees bent, and the hands behind the thighs. Shifting the weight back off of the sitting bones, balance with the spine, neck, and scapulae in neutral, and the feet off the floor. Extend the knees, keeping the hands behind the legs. Hold.

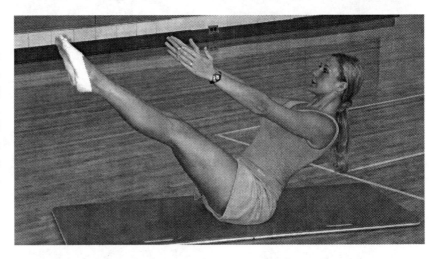

■ 9-4c. Standing bent-over row with weights:

Squat with the weight over the heels, the knees behind the toes, the tailbone pointing back, and the spine, neck, and scapulae in neutral. Hold completely stable, with the abdominals contracted, while performing a bilateral row with weights. The shoulders and elbows are the only moving joints.

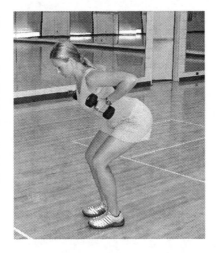
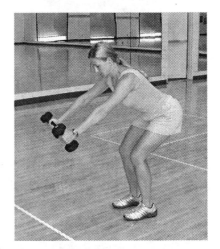

LEVEL 5: Multi-Muscle Groups with Increased Resistance and Core Challenge

■ **9-5a. Supine curl-up (spinal flexion) into a V-sit:**

Start in a supine position, with the knees bent. Perform spinal flexion, with the arms at the sides, all the way up into a V-sit position, with a neutral spine and neck, as previously described, and the knees extended. Balance, pause, and then roll back down through spinal flexion, completely articulating the spine back to neutral.

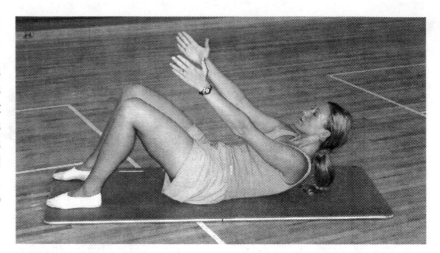

■ **9-5b. V-sit with a medicine ball rotation:**

Start in a V-sit, holding the medicine ball at chest height. Keeping the spine, neck, and scapulae in neutral, slowly rotate to one side, and then the other. Increase the level of difficulty of the exercise by holding the ball farther from the body.

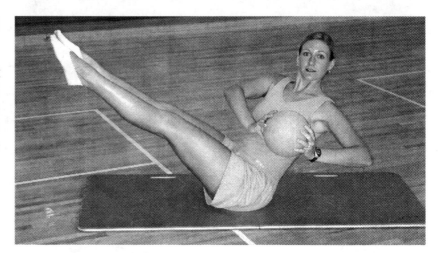

LEVEL 6: Add Balance, Increased Function, Speed, and/or Rotation

■ **9-6a. Stability ball walk-out, one leg balance:**

Lying in a prone position over the ball, "walk-out" until the ball is under the shoelaces. Maintain the spine, neck, pelvis, and scapulae in neutral. Keep the knees straight and the abdominals contracted. Balance on one leg.

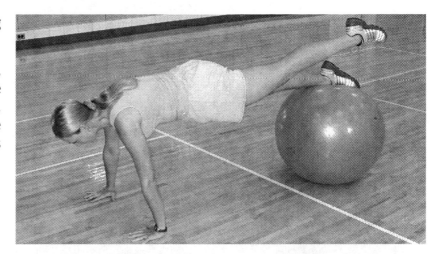

■ **9-6b. Stability ball elbow balance:**

Lying in a prone position with the abdominals on the ball, press up onto the elbows and lift the torso off the ball. Balance on the elbows and toes, with the abdominals contracted and the scapulae depressed and in neutral.

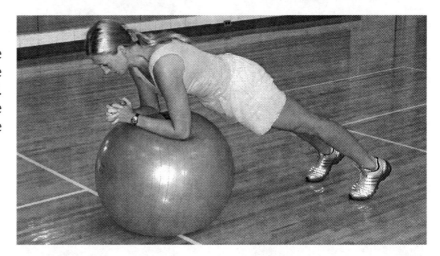

■ **9-6c. Standing lunge twist to balance:**

Start the exercise standing on one leg with one knee lifted, holding the medicine ball in front of the chest. Perform a back lunge, while simultaneously twisting to the same side, holding the ball away from the chest. Return to the starting position and repeat the exercise on the other side. Keep the spine, neck, pelvis, and scapulae completely neutral throughout the entire exercise. Maintain abdominal contraction.

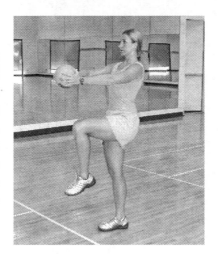
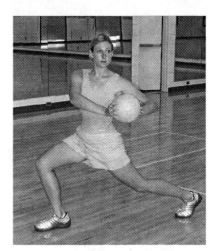

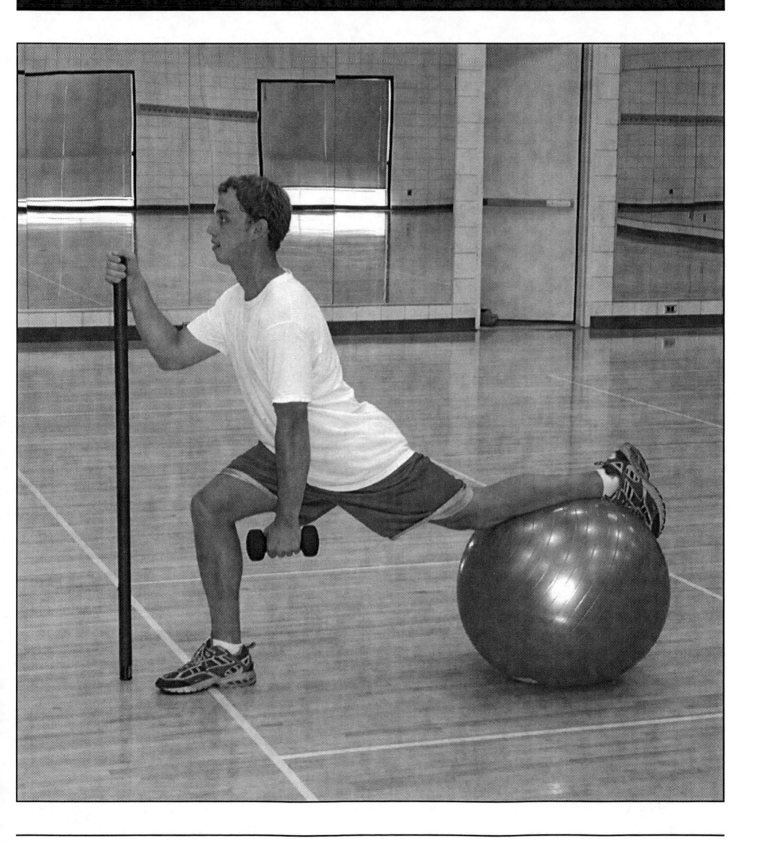

CHAPTER TEN
Quadriceps/Hip Flexors

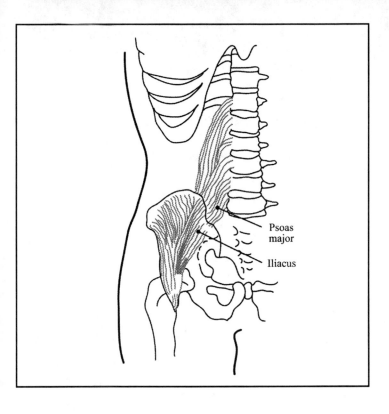

ILIOPSOAS

Primary Joint Actions:

- Hip flexion
- Anterior pelvic tilt

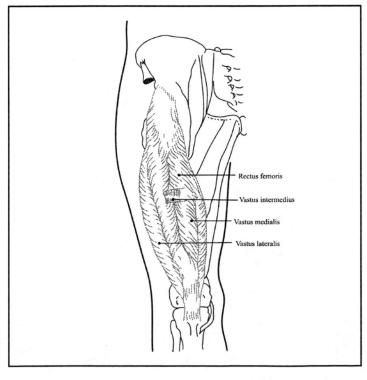

QUADRICEPS

Primary Joint Actions:

- Rectus Femoris

  √ Hip flexion

  √ Knee extension

- Vastus Lateralis

  √ Knee extension

- Vastus Intermedius

  √ Knee extension

- Vastus medialis

  √ Knee extension

LEVEL 1: Isolate/Educate

■ **10-1a. Seated quad sets:**

Sit with a rolled up towel or a blanket under one knee, maintaining good neutral spinal alignment, with the weight on the sitting bones, and the neck in line with the spine. Fully extend the working knee, firmly contracting the quadriceps muscles without using momentum.

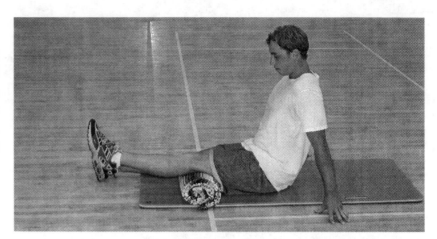

■ **10-1b. Supine unilateral knee extension /hip flexion:**

Lie in a supine position with the support knee bent, the spine, pelvis, and neck in neutral, and the abdominals engaged. Maintaining the working thigh at a 45° angle, slowly extend the knee, contracting the quadriceps. If performing hip flexion, start with the working leg on the floor; then flex the hip to a 45° angle and lower back to the starting position, maintaining torso stability.

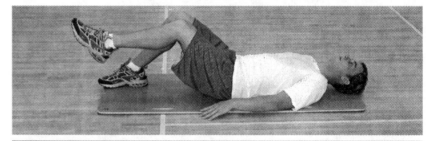

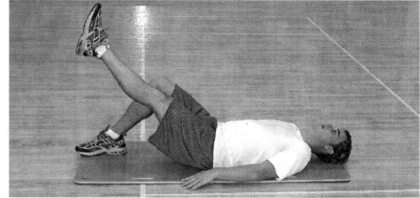

■ **10-1c. Seated unilateral knee extension:**

Sitting on a bench in good alignment, with the spine, pelvis, neck, and scapulae in neutral, slowly extend the working knee through its full range of motion. Firmly contract the quadriceps, gently tightening the kneecap.

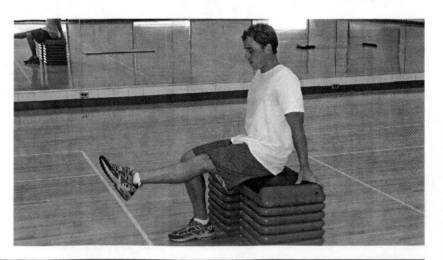

LEVEL 2: Isolate/Educate with Resistance

■ **10-2a. Supine unilateral knee extension/hip flexion with band:**

Lie in a supine position with the support knee bent, the spine, pelvis, and neck in neutral, the abdominals engaged, and an elastic band around the ankles. Maintaining the working thigh at a 45° angle, slowly extend the knee, contracting the quadriceps. If performing hip flexion, start with the working leg on the floor; then flex the hip to a 45° angle and lower back to the starting position, maintaining torso stability.

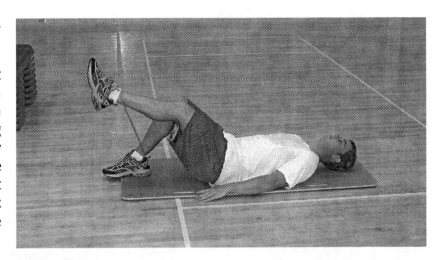

■ **10-2b. Seated unilateral knee extension with an elastic band:**

Sitting on a bench in good alignment, with the spine, pelvis, neck, and scapulae in neutral, and an elastic band around the ankles, slowly extend the working knee through its full range of motion. Firmly contract the quadriceps, gently tightening the kneecap.

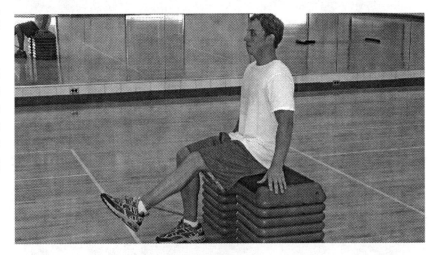

■ **10-2c. Badger knee extension VR machine:**

Sit on the machine in good alignment, with the pelvis, spine, scapulae, and neck in neutral, the abdominals engaged, and the knees level with cam. Smoothly extend the knees through the full range of motion without momentum, firmly contracting the quadriceps.

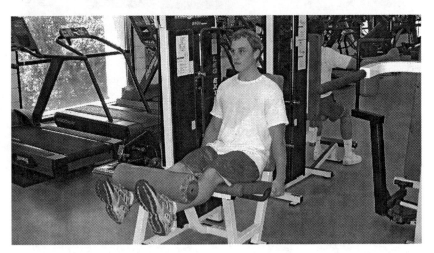

LEVEL 3: Add Functional Training Positions

■ **10-3a. Seated knee extension on a stability ball:**

Sit on the ball in good alignment, with the pelvis, spine, scapulae, and neck in neutral, and the body's weight on the sitting bones (ischial tuberosities). Keeping the hips level and the torso stable, extend the working knee, engaging the quadriceps.

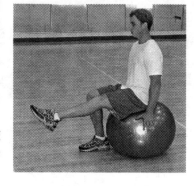

■ **10-3b. Wall squat with a stability ball:**

Stand with the ball against the wall at approximately low-back height, with the pelvis, spine, scapulae, and neck in neutral alignment. Position the feet far enough away from the wall so that the knees bend no greater than 90° when squat--ting; the feet are shoulder-width apart, with the knees in the same direction as the second toes. When squatting, do not allow the hips to drop below the knees.

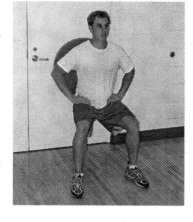

■ **10-3c. Squat with unilateral counterbalance arms:**

Stand with the feet hip or shoulder-width apart, and the pelvis, spine, scapulae, and neck in neutral alignment. Squat, hinging at the hips, maintaining the pelvis, spine, and neck in neutral, while contracting the abdominals. Shift the hips back so that the knees stay behind the toes. Alternate shoulder flexion for

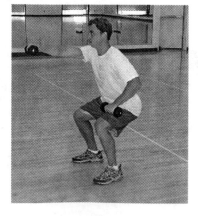

counterbalance, keeping one hand on the thigh for support and increased back safety.

■ **10-3d. Standing knee extension with bodybar support:**

Stand in good alignment, with the pelvis, spine, scapulae, and neck in neutral, the standing knee slightly flexed, the hips level, and the abdominals contracted, while holding the bar for balance. Flex the working hip and straighten and bend the working knee, contracting the quadriceps and the hip flexors. Maintain torso stability.

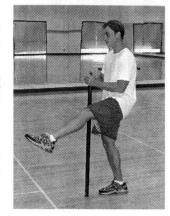

■ **10-3e. Standing knee extension on balance:**

Stand in good alignment, with the pelvis, spine, scapulae, and neck in neutral, the standing knee slightly flexed, the hips level, and the abdominals contracted. Flex the working hip and straighten and bend the working knee, contracting the quadriceps and the hip flexors. Maintain torso stability.

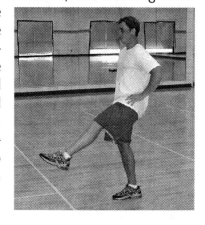

LEVEL 4: Combine Increased Function with Resistance

■ **10-4a. Seated knee extension on a stability ball with an elastic band:**

Sit on a ball in good alignment, with the pelvis, spine, scapulae, and neck in neutral, the body's weight on the sitting bones (ischial tuberosities), and an elastic band around the ankles. Keeping the hips level and the torso stable, extend the working knee, engaging the quadriceps.

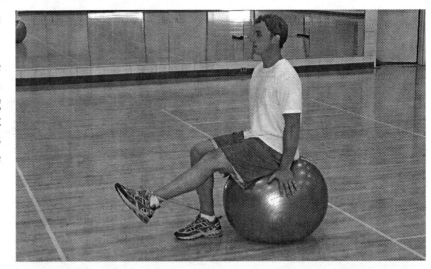

■ **10-4b. Standing knee extension on balance with an elastic band:**

Stand in good alignment, with the pelvis, spine, scapulae, and neck in neutral, the standing knee slightly flexed, the hips level, the abdominals contracted, and an elastic band around the ankles. Flex the working hip and straighten and bend the working knee, contracting the quadriceps and the hip flexors. Maintain torso stability.

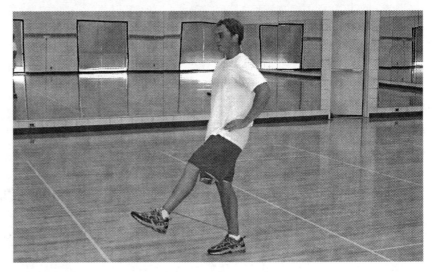

LEVEL 5: Multi-Muscle Groups with Increased Resistance and Core Challenge

■ **10-5a. Paramount leg press VR machine:**

Sit (or lie) on the machine with the pelvis, spine, scapulae, and neck in ideal alignment, the abdominals engaged, and the hips and knees flexed. Exhaling, smoothly extend the hips and knees, contracting the quadriceps, buttocks, and hamstrings.

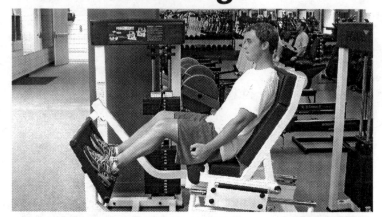

■ **10-5b. Modified squat (plie) with a dumbbell:**

Stand with the hips externally rotated (i.e., turned out), the toes lined up in the same direction as the knees, the feet wider than shoulder width, the pelvis, spine, scapulae, and neck in neutral, and the abdominals contracted. Hold the dumbbell with both hands. Bend both knees, pressing out in the direction of the second toes, taking care not to let the knees overshoot the toes (step laterally to put the feet farther apart if this happens). Return to the starting position, contracting the quadriceps, buttocks, hamstrings, and adductors.

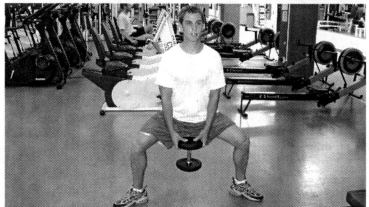

■ **10-5c. Smith machine squat:**

Stand with the feet hip or shoulder-width apart, slightly in front of the Smith machine, with the pelvis, spine, scapulae, and neck in neutral alignment. Squat, hinging at the hips, main-taining the pelvis, spine, and neck in neutral, while contracting the abdominals. Shift the hips and tailbone back so that the knees stay behind the toes. Return to the starting position, engaging the quadriceps, buttocks, and hamstrings. Maintain torso stability.

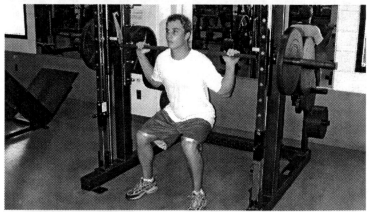

■ **10-5d. Smith machine squat on one leg:**

Stand with the feet hip or shoulder-width apart, slightly in front of a Smith machine, with the pelvis, spine, scapulae, and neck in neutral alignment. Squat, hinging at the hips, maintaining the pelvis, spine, and neck in neutral and contracting abdominals, with one hip flexed and one leg lifted. Shift the hips and tailbone back so that the support knee stays behind the toes.

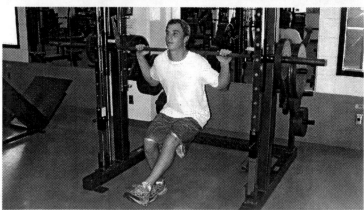

LEVEL 5: Multi-Muscle Groups with Increased Resistance and Core Challenge (cont'd)

■ **10-5e. Stationary lunge on a Smith machine:**

Stand under the bar with the feet staggered, maintain the back foot with the heel lifted, and the pelvis, spine, scapulae, and neck in neutral alignment. Keep the hips and shoulders level, and the abdominals contracted. Bend the knees and lower without moving or changing spinal alignment. Have the feet far enough apart so that the front knee stays behind the toes, and flexes no greater than 90°.

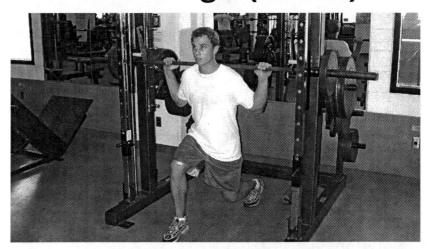

■ **10-5f. Front lunge with a barbell:**

Stand with the feet hip-width apart, the knees soft, the pelvis, spine, scapulae, and neck in neutral, and the bar across the shoulders (not on the vertebrae of the neck). Lunge forward, placing the foot far enough in front so that the knee does not bend greater than 90°, with the back heel off the floor, the hips and shoulders even and level, and the abdominals contracted. The back knee may be bent or straight (Note: a straight knee increases the difficulty of the exercise).

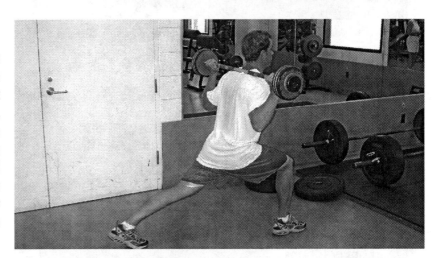

■ **10-5g. Free Motion squat/lift machine:**

Stand with the feet hip or shoulder-width apart, and the pelvis, spine, scapulae, and neck in neutral alignment, gripping the handles (or, alternatively, the dumbbells). Squat, hinging at the hips, maintaining the pelvis, spine, and neck, while contracting the abdominals. Shift the hips and tailbone back so that the knees stay behind the toes. Return to the starting position, engaging the quadriceps, buttocks, and hamstrings. Maintain torso stability.

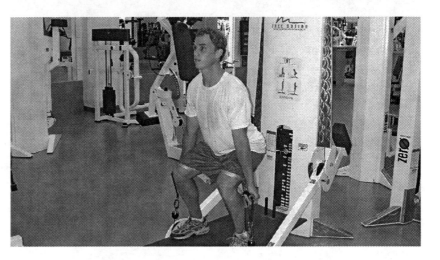

LEVEL 6: Add Balance, Increased Function, Speed, and/or Rotation

■ **10-6a. Squat to overhead press:**

Stand with the feet hip or shoulder-width apart, and the pelvis, spine, scapulae, and neck in neutral alignment; hold the bar across the shoulders, off the neck. Squat, hinging at the hips, maintaining the pelvis, spine, and neck in neutral, while contracting the abdominals. Shift the hips and tailbone back so that the knees stay behind the toes. Return to the starting position, engaging the quadriceps, buttocks, and hamstrings, while simultaneously pressing the bar up into an overhead press. Maintain torso stability.

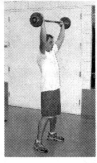
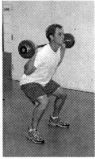

■ **10-6b. Slideboard lunge with weights:**

Place a slide bootie on the moving foot; keep the stationary foot off the slide. For a front lunge, stand at the back end of the slide; for a back lunge, stand at the front end. Start with the knees soft, the pelvis, spine, scapulae, and neck in neutral, and the abdominals engaged. Lunge, ensuring that the front knee does not bend greater than 90°, keeping the back heel off the floor, and the hips and shoulders even and level; hold

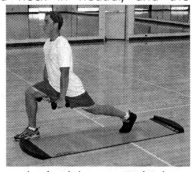

the weights at the sides. The back knee may be bent or straight (Note: a straight knee increases the difficulty of the exercise).

■ **10-6c. Split lunge on a stability ball:**

Stand with the back foot centered on the stability ball, with the same-side hand holding the dumbbell, and the opposite-side hand on the bar or wall for

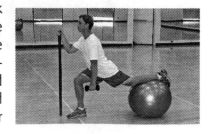

support. Keeping the pelvis, spine, scapulae, and neck in neutral throughout, lunge, while rolling the back foot backwards on the ball, flexing the front knee no greater than 90°. Keep the hips and shoulders level and squared, and the abdominals engaged.

■ **10-6d. "Russian" traveling lunges:**

Start in a balanced "crane" position, with the left knee and hip flexed, the right knee soft, the pelvis, spine, scapulae, and neck in neutral, the abdominals engaged, and the elbows flexed, while holding weights at shoulder height. Under control, extend the left knee and lunge the left foot far forward (the knee flexes no greater than 90°), while simultaneously performing an overhead press. Move forwards to a standing position, subsequently lifting the right knee into the "crane" position.

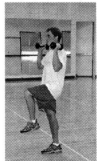
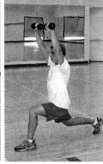

■ **10-6e. Plyometric lunges:**

Stand in a lunge position, with the feet staggered, the knees soft, the pelvis, spine, scapulae, and neck in neutral, the back heel off the floor, and the abdominals engaged. Springing upwards, switch legs in mid-air, landing softly under control, with the front knee flexing no greater than 90°. The back knee may be bent or straight (note: the straighter the back leg, the greater the difficulty of the exercise). Be cautious when adding dumbbells to increase the level of resistance.

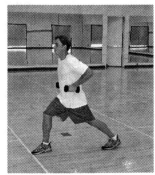

CHAPTER ELEVEN

Hamstrings and Buttocks

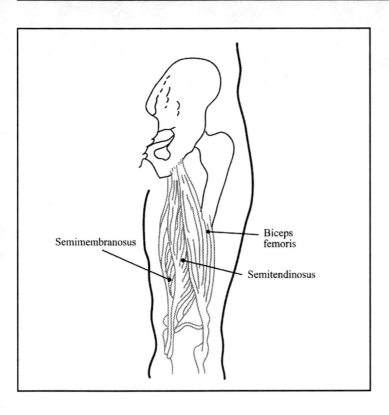

Semimembranosus

Biceps femoris

Semitendinosus

HAMSTRINGS

Primary Joint Actions:

- Hip extension
- Knee flexion

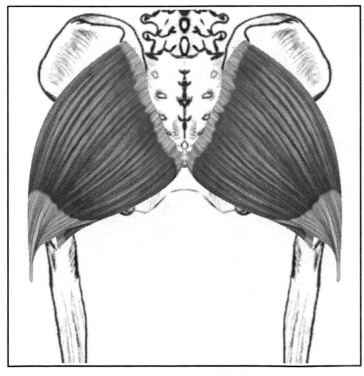

GLUTEUS MAXIMUS

Primary Joint Actions:

- Hip extension
- Hip outward rotation

LEVEL 1: Isolate/Educate

■ **11-1a. Supine buttock squeezes:**

Lie in a supine position with the knees bent, the feet flat on the floor, the pelvis, spine, scapulae, and neck in neutral, and the abdominals contracted. Squeeze the buttock (gluteal) muscles, keeping the mid-back on floor, while exhaling.

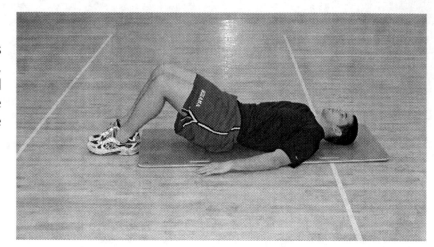

■ **11-1b. Prone hip extension, alternated with knee flexion:**

Lie in a prone position with the pelvis and spine in neutral, the neck in line with the spine, and the forehead down. Keep the hips down and level, and the abdominals contracted. Engaging the glutes and hamstrings, extend the working leg and then perform knee flexion. Return to the starting position, keeping the hips level and the back still.

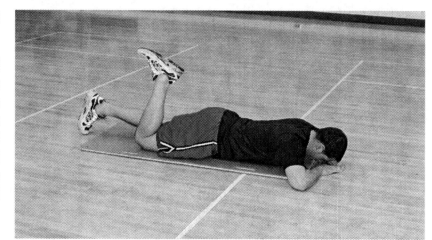

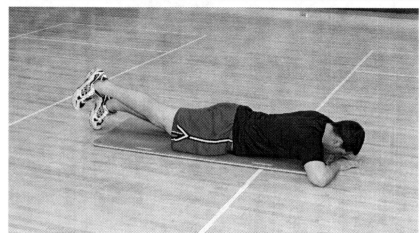

LEVEL 2: Isolate/Educate with Resistance

■ **11-2a. Prone hip extension, alternated with knee flexion, using an elastic band:**

Lie in a prone position with the pelvis and spine in neutral, the neck in line with the spine, the forehead down, and an elastic band around the ankles. Keep the hips down and level, and the abdominals contracted. Engaging the glutes and hamstrings, extend the working hip, then perform knee flexion, and then return to the starting position, keeping the hips level and the back still.

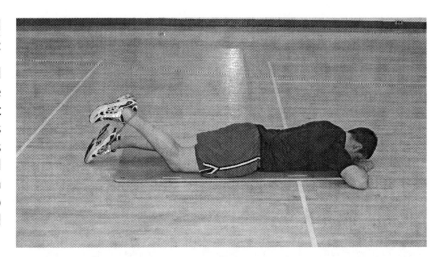

■ **11-2b. Badger seated leg curl VR machine:**

Sit on the machine with the knees aligned with the cam, the pelvis, spine, scapulae, and neck in neutral, and the abdominals engaged. Flex the knees, contracting the hamstrings; maintain a stable torso.

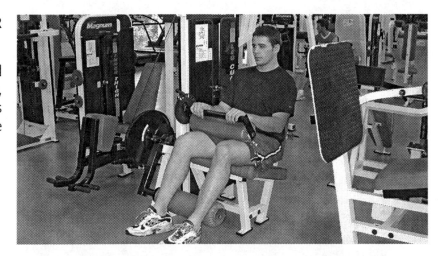

■ **11-2c. Paramount prone leg curl VR machine:**

Lie in a prone position on the machine, with the pelvis, spine, scapulae, and neck in neutral. Keeping the hips down and level and the abdominals engaged, flex the knees and curl the pad towards the buttocks, contracting the hamstrings.

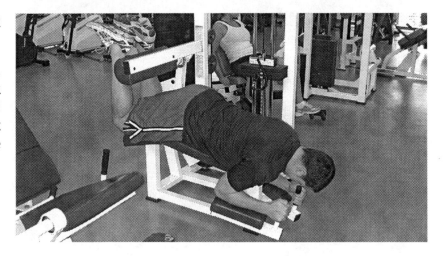

LEVEL 3: Add Functional Training Positions

■ **11-3a. All fours hip extension and knee flexion:**

On the elbows and knees, place the pelvis and spine in neutral and keep the head and neck in line with the spine, while pulling the abdominals upward. Perform hip extension and knee flexion, while keeping the hips perfectly level and the spine completely still, engaging the hamstrings and the buttocks throughout.

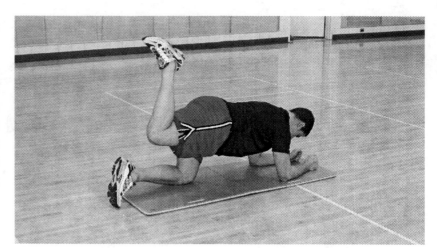

■ **11-3b. Standing hip extension/knee flexion with bodybar support:**

Stand on one foot, with the support knee soft, the pelvis, spine, scapulae, and neck in neutral, and the abdominals engaged. Hold the bodybar, barre, or wall for support. Press the moving leg backwards into hip extension and/or knee flexion, while keeping the hips level and the back and torso quite still.

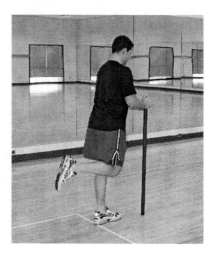
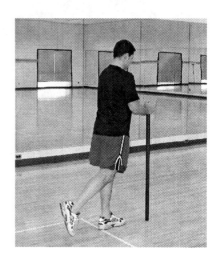

LEVEL 4: Combine Increased Function with Resistance

■ **11-4a. Standing balance hip extension/knee flexion, with an elastic band:**

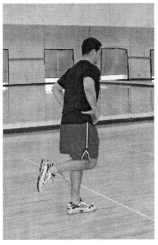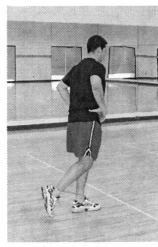

Stand on one foot, with the support knee soft, the pelvis, spine, scapulae, and neck in neutral, the abdominals engaged, and an elastic band around the ankles. Press the moving leg backwards into hip extension and/or knee flexion, while keeping the hips level and the back and torso quite still.

■ **11-4b. Supine knee flexion with a stability ball:**

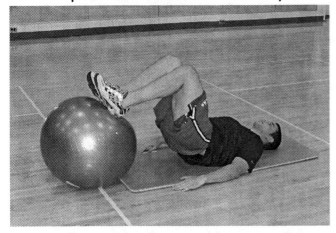

Lie in a supine position, with the heels on a stability ball. Lift up into a reverse plank and maintain the pelvis and spine in neutral, the buttocks and abdominals engaged, and the neck extended and relaxed on the floor. Keeping the hips level, flex the knees and roll the ball towards the buttocks using the heels, engaging the hamstrings. Straighten the legs out, maintaining a reverse plank and a stable torso.

■ **11-4c. Paramount standing hip extension VR machine:**

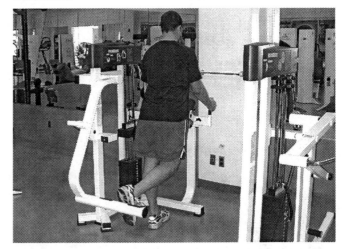

Stand on one foot, with the support knee soft, the pelvis, spine, scapulae, and neck in neutral, the abdominals engaged, and the hips pressed against the pad. Press the moving leg backwards into hip extension and/or knee flexion, while keeping the hips level and the back and torso quite still.

■ **11-4d. Standing hip extension/knee flexion at a low pulley:**

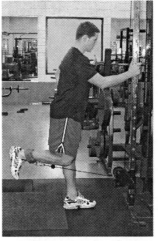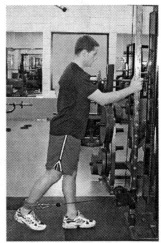

Stand on one foot, with the support knee soft, the pelvis, spine, scapulae, and neck in neutral, the abdominals engaged, and a cuff around the ankle. Press the moving leg backwards into hip extension and/or knee flexion, while keeping the hips level and the back and torso quite still. Progress to performing this exercise without the support of the hands.

LEVEL 5: Multi-Muscle Groups with Increased Resistance and Core Challenge

■ **11-5a. Standing hip extension, with an elastic band and front raises:**

Stand on one foot, with the support knee soft, the pelvis, spine, scapulae, and neck in neutral, the abdominals engaged, and an elastic band around the ankles. Press the moving leg backwards into hip extension, keeping the hips level and the back and torso quite still. Simultaneously perform bilateral front raises, keeping the scapulae down and the neck extended.

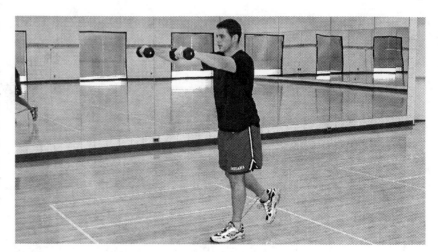

■ **11-5b. Standing hip extension, with an elastic band and lateral raises:**

Stand on one foot, with the support knee soft, the pelvis, spine, scapulae, and neck in neutral, the abdominals engaged, and an elastic band around the ankles. Press the moving leg backwards into hip extension, keeping the hips level and the back and torso quite still. Simultaneously perform lateral raises, keeping the scapulae down, the neck extended, the wrists straight, and the elbows slightly flexed.

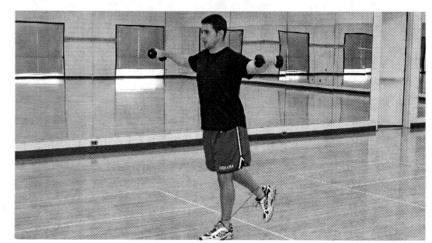

LEVEL 6: Add Balance, Increased Function, Speed, and/or Rotation

■ 11-6a. Back lunge on a slideboard:

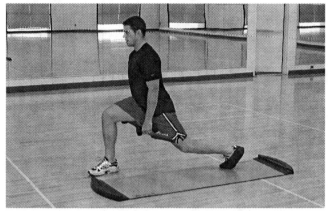

Place a slide bootie on the moving foot; keep the stationary foot off the slide. Standing at the front end of the slideboard, start with the knees soft, the pelvis, spine, scapulae, and neck in neutral, and the abdominals engaged. Lunge back on the slide, ensuring that the front knee does not bend greater than 90°, keeping the back heel off the floor, and the hips and shoulders even and level, while holding weights at the sides. The back knee may be bent or straight (note: a straight knee increases the level of difficulty of the exercise).

■ 11-6b. Prone hip extension on a stability ball with partner resistance:

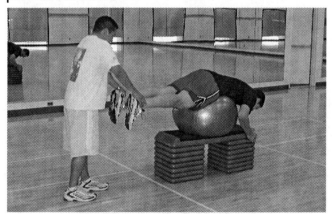

Place a stability ball on a bench; lie in a prone position over the bench with a stability ball under the lower abdominals and hips; grasp the bench. Keeping the pelvis, spine, scapulae, and neck in neutral and the hips even, perform bilateral hip extension, engaging the hamstrings and buttocks, against the partner's resistance.

■ 11-6c. Good mornings with a barbell:

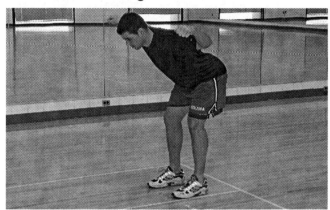

Stand in good alignment, with a barbell across the shoulders, the knees soft, and the pelvis, spine, and neck in neutral. Hinging at the hips, maintain a perfectly neutral spine and a stable torso, with the abdominals fully engaged, and the tailbone pointing back. Return to the starting position, contracting the buttocks, hamstrings, and core muscles. Note: this exercise involves a relatively higher level of risk; it is appropriate only for those individuals who have no history of back pain and who have excellent core stability and hamstring/low-back flexibility.

■ 11-6d. One-leg balance hip extension with floor touch:

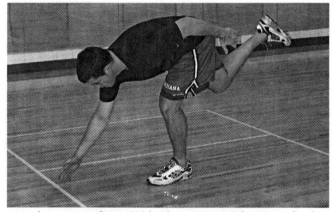

Stand on one foot, with the support knee soft, the pelvis, spine, scapulae, and neck in neutral, and the abdominals engaged. Press the moving leg backwards into hip extension and/or knee flexion, while simultaneously hip hinging and reaching towards the floor. Maintain core stability throughout.

CHAPTER TWELVE

Gluteus Medius

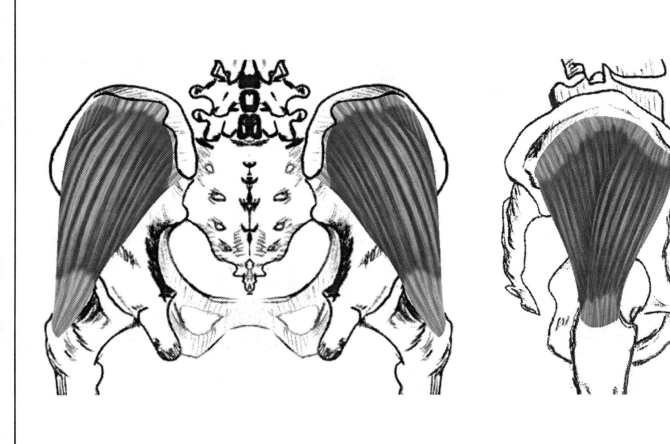

GLUTEUS MEDIUS

Primary Joint Action:

- Hip abduction

LEVEL 1: Isolate/Educate

■ **12-1a. Side-lying abduction, short lever:**

Lie on the side, with the hips and shoulders stacked, the pelvis, spine, and neck in neutral, the abdominals contracted, the hips flexed approximately at a 45° angle, and the knees flexed. Slowly abduct the hip, engaging the gluteus medius.

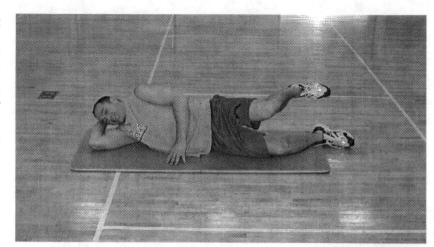

■ **12-1b. Side-lying abduction, short lever with rotation variation:**

Lie on the side, with the hips and shoulders stacked, the pelvis, spine, and neck in neutral, the abdominals contracted, the hips flexed approximately at a 45° angle, and the knees flexed. Slowly abduct and externally rotate the hip, engaging the gluteus medius.

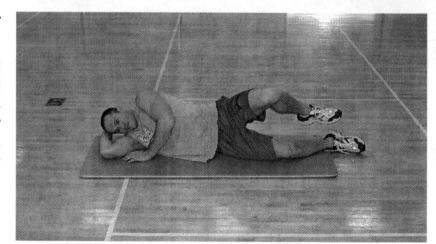

■ **12-1c. Side-lying abduction, long lever:**

Lie on the side with the hips and shoulders stacked, the pelvis, spine, and neck in neutral, the abdominals contracted, the hips flexed approximately at a 45° angle, and the knees straight. Slowly abduct the hip, engaging the gluteus medius.

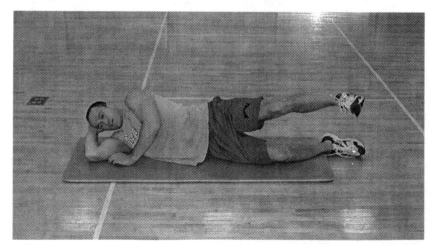

LEVEL 2: Isolate/Educate with Resistance

■ **12-2a. Badger seated hip abduction VR machine:**

Sit on the machine with the pelvis, spine, scapulae, and neck in neutral, and the abdominals contracted. Engaging the hip abductors, perform bilateral hip abduction.

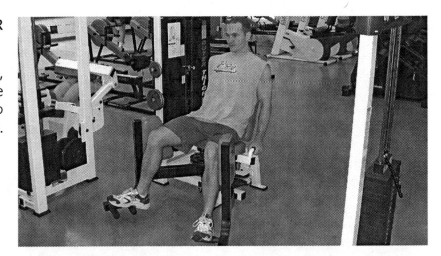

■ **12-2b. Side-lying abduction, with an elastic band:**

Lie on the side, with the hips and shoulders stacked, the pelvis, spine, and neck in neutral, the abdominals contracted, the hips flexed approximately at a 45° angle, the knees straight or bent, and an elastic band just above the knees. Slowly abduct the hip, engaging the gluteus medius.

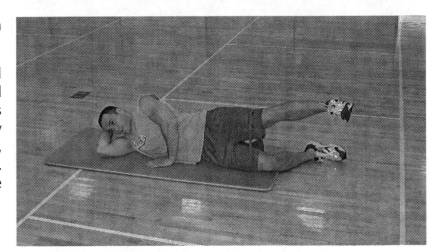

LEVEL 3: Add Functional Training Positions

■ **12-3a. All fours hip abduction, with an elastic band:**

On the hands and knees, place the pelvis, spine, scapulae, and neck in neutral, contract the abdominals, and square the hips and shoulders. With an elastic band around the thighs just above the knees, perform hip abduction, keeping the torso completely still. The knee brushes out to the side (abduction), rather than lifting up (involves spinal rotation).

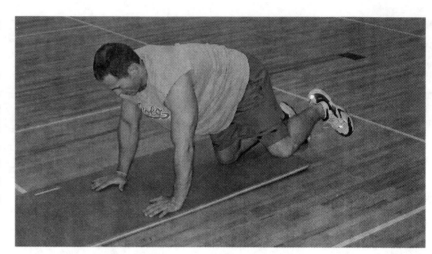

■ **12-3b. Standing abduction, with an elastic band and with bodybar support:**

Stand on one foot, with the support knee soft, the pelvis, spine, scapulae, and neck in good alignment, the hips and shoulders square and level, the abdominals engaged, and the hands on a bodybar (or barre or wall) for support. Abduct the hip, keeping the kneecap facing front, the hips square, and the torso completely still.

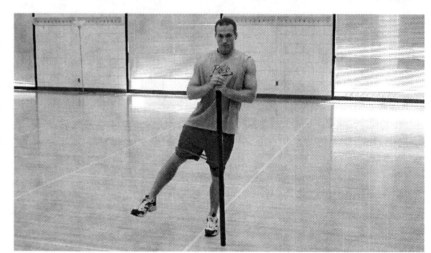

■ **12-3c. Badger standing multi-hip VR machine:**

Stand on the machine platform, with the support knee soft, the pelvis, spine, scapulae, and neck in good alignment, the hips and shoulders square and level, the abdominals engaged, the hands on the hand rests, and the pad against the thigh. Abduct the hip, keeping the kneecap facing front, the hips square, and the torso completely still.

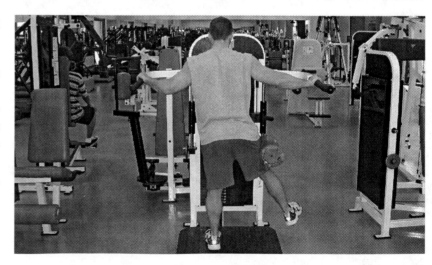

LEVEL 4: Combine Increased Function with Resistance

■ **12-4a. Standing alternating hip abduction, with an elastic band:**

Stand with the feet hip-width apart, the knees soft, the pelvis, spine, scapulae, and neck in neutral, the abdominals engaged, and an elastic band around the thighs just above the knees. Abduct the hip on one side and then on the other, keeping the pelvis squared, level, and still. Maintain a stable torso throughout.

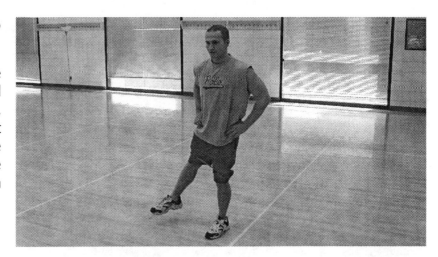

■ **12-4b. Standing hip abduction, with a low pulley:**

Stand on one foot, with the support knee soft, facing sideways to the pulley unit, with a cuff around the outside ankle, the pelvis, spine, scapulae, and neck in good alignment, the hips and shoulders square and level, and the abdominals engaged. Abduct the hip, keeping the kneecap facing front, the hips square, and the torso completely still while balancing.

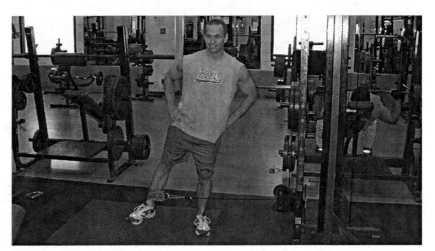

LEVEL 5: Multi-Muscle Groups with Increased Resistance and Core Challenge

■ **12-5a. Squat to hip abduction, with biceps curls:**

Stand with the feet shoulder-width apart, the knees soft, the pelvis, spine, scapulae, and neck in neutral, and the abdominals contracted, holding dumbbells. Perform a standard weightroom squat, hinging at hips, with the tailbone back, the spine in neutral, the abdominals contracted, and the knees behind the toes. Return to the starting position and simultaneously perform hip abduction and a bilateral biceps curl, keeping the hips square and the knee facing forwards. Squat, and repeat on the other side.

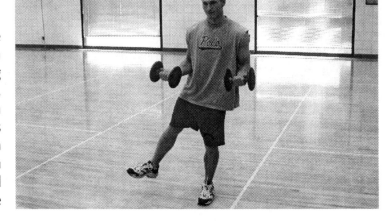

■ **12-5b. Squat to hip abduction with an elastic band, lateral raise with dumbbells**

Stand holding dumbbells, with the feet shoulder-width apart, the knees soft, the pelvis, spine, scapulae, and neck in neutral, the abdominals contracted, and an elastic band around the thighs. Perform a standard weightroom squat, hinging at the hips, with the tailbone back, the spine in neutral, the abdominals contracted, and the knees behind the toes. Return to the starting position and simultaneously perform hip abduction and a lateral raise, keeping the hips square and the knee facing forwards. Squat, and repeat on the other side.

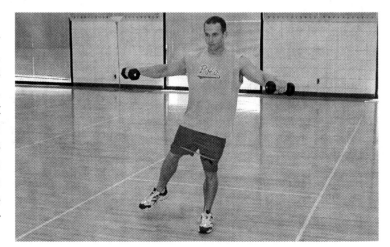

■ **12-5c. Side lunge with a unilateral front raise:**

Stand holding a dumbbell in the left hand, with the feet shoulder-width apart, the knees soft, the pelvis, spine, scapulae, and neck in neutral, and the abdominals contracted. Abduct the right leg, moving into a side lunge on the right side, with the right knee bent at a 90° angle, the hip hinging, the tailbone back, the spine in neutral, the abdominals lifted, and the right hand on the thigh. Simultaneously, perform a front raise with the left arm, providing a counterbalance. To return, push off with the right foot, lift the leg back into hip abduction, and bring the leg back. Repeat on the same side 8-12 times.

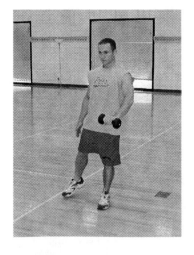
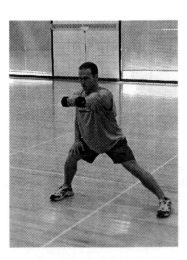

LEVEL 6: Add Balance, Increased Function, Speed, and/or Rotation

■ **12-6a. Side-lying hip abduction on a stability ball:**

Perform a side plank, with a stability ball under the lower ribs and waist, the hips and shoulders stacked, the pelvis, spine, and neck in neutral, and the abdominals engaged, while lying on the side of the bottom foot (alternatively, the bottom knee can be placed on the floor). Maintaining a stable position, abduct the top hip, contracting the gluteus medius.

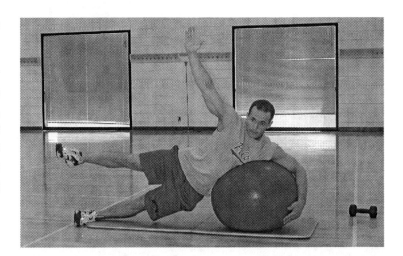

■ **12-6b. Standing 4-count hip abduction, with an overhead press:**

Stand on one foot holding dumbbells in front of the shoulders with the elbows flexed, with the support knee soft, the pelvis, spine, scapulae, and neck in good alignment, the hips and shoulders square and level, and the abdominals engaged. Perform hip abduction with four small pulses, lifting higher with each count, keeping the kneecap facing front, the hips square, and the torso completely still. Simultaneously perform a bilateral overhead press. Repeat on the other side.

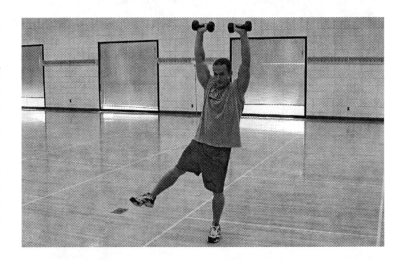

■ **12-6c. Standing unilateral hip abduction, with medial/lateral rotation and lateral raise:**

Stand on one foot, holding a dumbbell in the left hand, with the support knee soft, the pelvis, spine, scapulae, and neck in good alignment, the hips and shoulders square and level, and the abdominals engaged. Perform hip abduction with the right leg; hold and balance while laterally rotating; then medially rotate the right hip and simultaneously perform a lateral raise with the left arm.

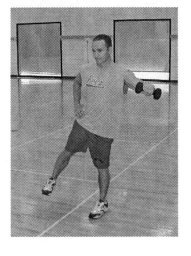
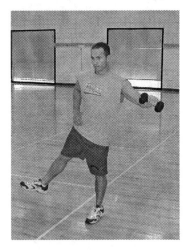

CHAPTER THIRTEEN

Adductors

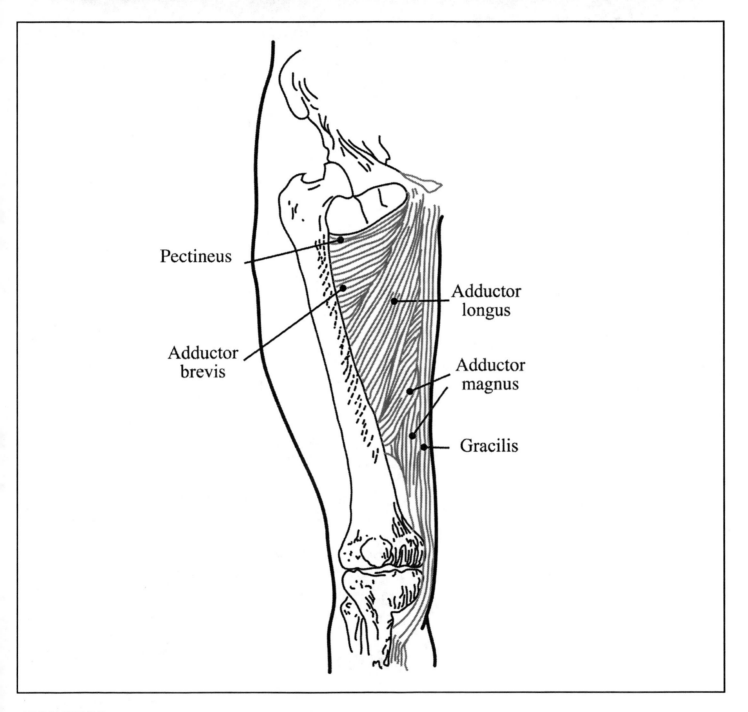

Pectineus

Adductor longus

Adductor brevis

Adductor magnus

Gracilis

ADDUCTORS

Primary Joint Action:

- Hip adduction

LEVEL 1: Isolate/Educate

■ **13-1a. Side-lying, short-lever adduction:**

Lie on the side, with the hips and shoulders stacked, the spine and neck in neutral, the top hand on the floor for support, and the abdominals contracted. Place the top leg in front, with the side of the foot on the floor; keep the top knee slightly elevated to maintain stacked hips (a step, pad, or pillow may be used if necessary). Adduct the bottom leg with the knee bent (a short lever), engaging the inner thigh muscles. Keep the head in line with the spine.

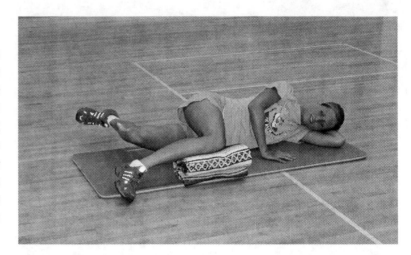

■ **13-1b. Side-lying, long-lever adduction:**

Lie on the side, with the hips and shoulders stacked, the spine and neck in neutral, the top hand on the floor for support, and the abdominals contracted. Place the top leg in front, with the side of the foot on the floor; keep the top knee slightly elevated to maintain stacked hips (a step, pad, or pillow may be used if necessary). Adduct the bottom leg with the knee straight (a long lever), engaging the inner thigh muscles. Keep the head in line with the spine.

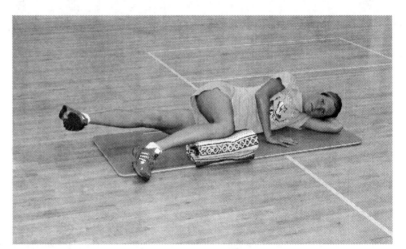

■ **13-1c. Supine long-lever adduction:**

Lie on the back, with the spine and neck in neutral, and the torso stabilized. Flex the hips to approximately a 90° angle; keep the knees slightly flexed for a long lever (a short-lever adduction may be performed by those individuals who have limited hamstring flexibility). Open the thighs to about shoulder-width apart, squeezing the adductors on the return.

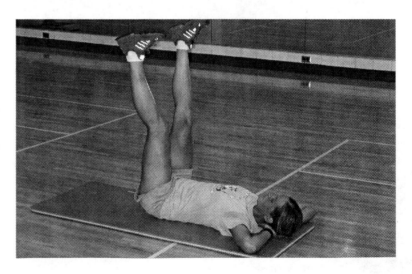

LEVEL 2: Isolate/Educate with Resistance

■ **13-2a. Side-lying, short-lever adduction with manual resistance:**

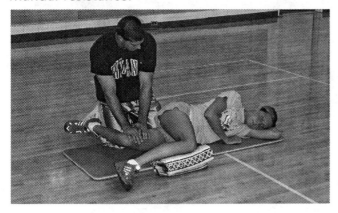

Lie on the side, with the hips and shoulders stacked, the spine and neck in neutral, the top hand on the floor for support, and the abdominals contracted. Place the top leg in front, with the side of the foot on the floor for support, and the abdominals contracted. Keep the top knee slightly elevated to maintain stacked hips (a step, pad, or pillow may be used if necessary). Adduct the bottom leg with the knee bent (a short lever), engaging the inner thigh muscles, against the partner's manual resistance. Keep the head in line with the spine.

■ **13-2b. Side-lying, long-lever adduction with a Body Bar:**

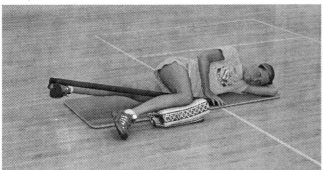

Lie on the side with the hips and shoulders stacked, the spine and neck in neutral, the top hand on the floor for support, and the abdominals contracted. Place the top leg in front, with the side of the foot on the floor; keep the top knee slightly elevated to maintain stacked hips (a step, pad, or pillow may be used if necessary). Adduct the bottom leg with the knee bent (a short lever), engaging the inner thigh muscles, against the BodyBar. Keep the head in line with the spine.

■ **13-2c. Supine adduction with a stability ball:**

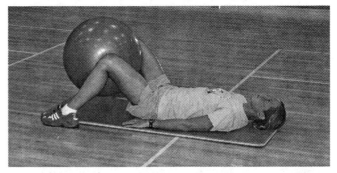

Lie on the back, with the spine and neck in neutral, the torso stabilized, the knees bent, and the feet on the floor. With a ball between the thighs, adduct the hips, engaging the inner thigh muscles. Keep the abdominals contracted.

■ **13-2d. Badger seated hip adduction VR machine:**

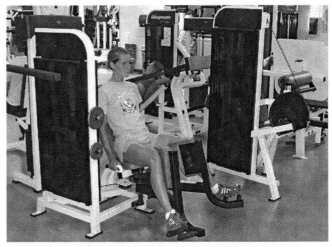

Sit in the hip adduction machine, with the spine, neck, and scapulae in neutral, and the abdominals contracted. Engaging the inner thigh muscles, adduct the hips. Slowly return.

LEVEL 3: Add Functional Training Positions

■ **13-3a. Standing plie with a stability ball:**

Stand in good alignment, with the feet shoulder-width apart, the hips externally rotated, the tailbone down, and the pelvis, spine, scapulae, and neck in neutral. Plie, flexing the knees, while maintaining the spine in neutral, with the tailbone down. Return to the starting position, squeezing the ball between the legs, thereby engaging the hip adductors.

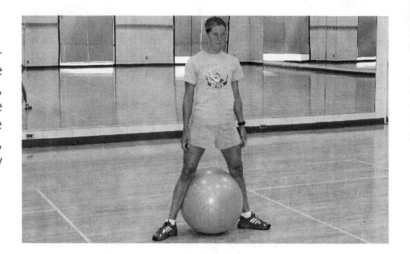

■ **13-3b. Standing hip adduction, with an elastic band, and with a Body Bar for support:**

Stand in good alignment, with the knees soft, the pelvis spine, scapulae, and neck in neutral, and an elastic band around the ankles. Hold a BodyBar for support. Balancing on one foot, contract the moving-side adductors and bring the foot in front of the support leg. Keep the hips level, the knees soft, and the torso stable throughout.

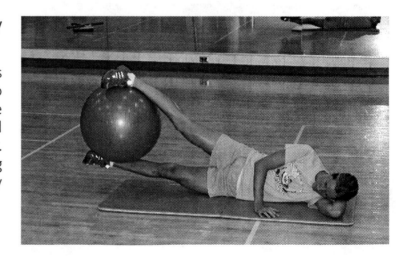

■ **13-3c. Side-lying adduction with a stability ball:**

Lie on the side, with the hips and shoulders stacked, the spine and neck in neutral, the top hand on the floor for support, and the abdominals contracted. Place a stability ball between the ankles; keep the legs straight. Perform hip adduction with the bottom leg, lifting both legs. Grip the ball with both legs by contracting the adductors.

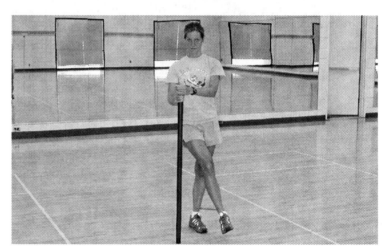

LEVEL 4: Combine Increased Function with Resistance

13-4a. Badger multi-hip VR machine:

Stand facing the multi-hip machine; adjust the cam to hip height and the pad to the middle of the inner thigh. Have the support knee soft, the pelvis, spine, neck, and scapulae in neutral, and the abdominals contracted. Perform hip adduction with the working leg, keeping the hips and shoulders level, and the torso perfectly stable throughout.

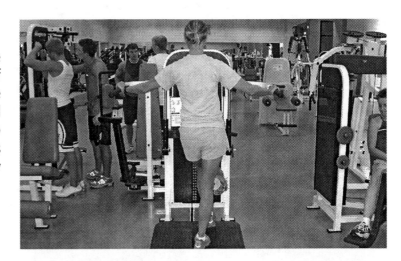

13-4b. Standing adduction at a low pulley, with support

Stand to the side of the low pulley with a cuff around the inside ankle. Keep the knees soft, the tailbone down, the pelvis, spine, scapulae, and neck in neutral, and the abdominals contracted. Hold onto the machine for support and externally rotate both legs. Adduct the working leg, bringing the leg slightly in front of the support leg and maintaining turnout to facilitate full adduction.

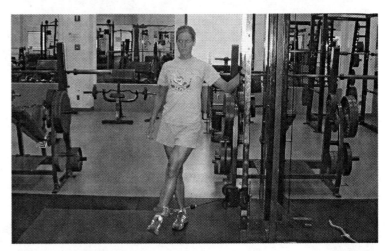

13-4c. Standing adduction at a low pulley, with no support:

Stand to the side of the low pulley with a cuff around the inside ankle. Keep the knees soft, the tailbone down, the pelvis, spine, scapulae, and neck in neutral, and the abdominals contracted. Balancing on the outside foot, externally rotate both legs. Adduct the working leg, bringing the leg slightly in front of the support leg and maintaining turnout to facilitate full adduction.

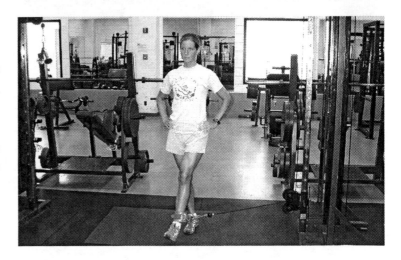

LEVEL 5: Multi-Muscle Groups with Increased Resistance and Core Challenge

■ **13-5a. Squat, with adductor drag:**

Step to the side while performing a standard squat, with the knees flexed no greater than a 90° angle, the knees behind the toes, the tailbone pointing back, the spine, neck, and scapulae in neutral, and the abdominals contracted. During the return to the starting (standing) position, perform hip adduction, while dragging the moving foot against the floor, returning the feet to hip-width apart, and contracting the adductors. Step out to the same side again, squat, and adduct and drag the moving leg again. Repeat 4-8 times to one side, and then 4-8 times to the other side.

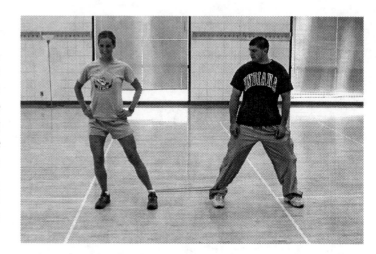

■ **13-5b. Supine adduction at a Smith machine, with curl-ups:**

Lie in a supine position on a mat in front of a Smith machine. Opening the legs, anchor each ankle to the stands with elastic tubing or bands. Place the pelvis, spine, neck, and scapulae in neutral; engage the abdominals to stabilize the torso. Adduct the inner thighs, while simultaneously performing abdominal curl-ups to approximately 30-40° of spinal flexion.

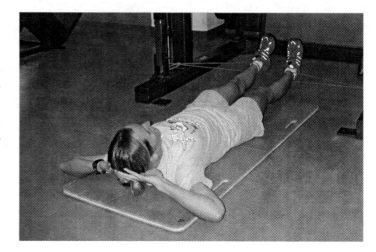

LEVEL 6: Add Balance, Increased Function, Speed, and/or Rotation

■ **13-6a. Side lunge on a slideboard, with balance:**

Place a slide bootie on the working-side foot; place the support foot on the floor near the end of the slide. Perform a side lunge with the working leg, sliding the foot along the slide; place the working-side hand on the thigh for support (the opposite arm may be counterbalanced in front, with a dumbbell, if desired). Keep the working-side knee behind the toes, the tailbone back (a squat position), the spine, neck, and scapulae in neutral, and the abdominals contracted. Return to the starting position by adducting the working-side leg, dragging the foot against the slideboard, until fully upright; pause and balance with the working-side leg slightly abducted. Repeat.

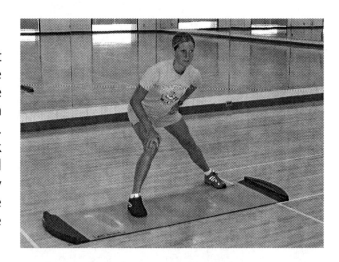

■ **13-6b. Bilateral adduction on a slideboard:**

With booties on both feet, stand in the middle of the slide, with the knees soft, and the pelvis, spine, neck, and scapulae in neutral. The hips may be externally rotated or neutral. Abduct the legs and slide back into the beginning stance, adducting the hips and engaging the inner thigh muscles on the return.

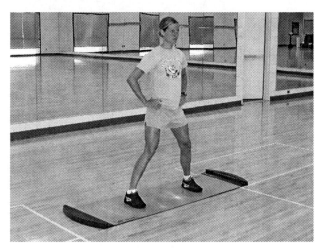

Shoulder Joint Muscles and their Actions

	Flexion	Extension	Abduction	Adduction	Internal Rotation	External Rotation	Horizontal Adduction	Horizontal Abduction
Anterior deltoid	PM		Asst		Asst		PM	
Medial deltoid			PM					PM
Posterior deltoid		Asst				Asst		PM
Supraspinatus			PM					
PecMajor, clav.	PM		Asst		Asst		PM	
PecMajor, stern		PM		PM	Asst		PM	
Subscapularis	Asst		Asst	Asst	PM		Asst	
Latissimus dorsi		PM		PM	Asst			Asst
Teres major		PM		PM	PM			Asst
Infraspinatus						PM		PM
Teres minor						PM		PM
Biceps,long head			Asst					
Biceps,short head	Asst			Asst	Asst		Asst	
Triceps,long head		Asst		Asst				

PM = Prime Mover   Asst = Assistant Mover

Shoulder Girdle Muscles and their Actions

	Elevation	Depression	Protraction	Retraction	Upward Rotation	Downward Rotation
Pectoralis minor		PM	PM			PM
Serratus anterior			PM		PM	
Trapezius I	PM					
Trapezius II	PM			Asst	PM	
Trapezius III				PM		
Trapezius IV		PM		Asst	PM	
Levator scapulae	PM					
Rhomboids	PM			PM		PM

PM = Prime Mover   Asst = Assistant Mover

Elbow Joint Muscles and their Actions

	Flexion	Extension	Pronation	Supination
Biceps brachii	PM			Asst
Brachialis	PM			
Brachioradialis	PM		Asst*	Asst*
Pronator teres	Asst		Asst	
Pronator quadratus			PM	
Triceps brachii		PM		
Anconeus		Asst		
Supinator				PM

PM = Prime Mover   Asst = Assistant Mover   * To the mid position

Knee Joint Muscles and their Actions

	Flexion	Extension	Inward Rotation	Outward Rotation
Biceps femoris	PM		PM	
Semitendinosus	PM		PM	
Semimembranosus	PM			PM
Rectus femoris		PM		
Vastus lateralis		PM		
Vastus intermedius		PM		
Vastus medialis		PM		
Sartorius	Asst		Asst	
Gracilis	Asst		Asst	
Popliteus	Asst		PM	
Gastrocnemius	Asst			

PM = Prime Mover   Asst = Assistant Mover

Hip Joint Muscles and their Actions

	Flexion	Extension	Abduction	Adduction	Inward Rotation	Outward Rotation
Psoas	PM		Asst			Asst
Iliacus	PM		Asst			Asst
Sartorius	Asst		Asst			Asst
Rectus femoris	PM		Asst			
Pectineus	PM			PM	Asst	
Gluteus maximus		PM	Asst*	Asst+		PM
Gluteus minimus	Asst~	Asst*	Asst		PM	Asst*
Gluteus medius	Asst~	Asst*	PM		Asst~	Asst*
Tensor fasciae latae	Asst		Asst		Asst	
Biceps femoris		PM				Asst
Semitendinosus		PM			Asst	
Semimembranosus		PM			Asst	
Gracilis	Asst			PM	Asst	
Adductor longus	Asst			PM	Asst	
Adductor brevis	Asst			PM	Asst	
Adductor magnus	Asst*	Asst+		PM	Asst	
Six outward rotators						PM

PM = Prime Mover   Asst = Assistant Mover   *Upper fibers   +Lower fibers   ~Anterior fibers

Bibliography

Kinesiology, 7th Ed. Luttgens K., Wells K.F. WB Saunders Pub., Philadelphia, PA, 1982.

Brunnstrom's Clinical Kinesiology, 4th Ed. Lehmkuhl L.D., Smith L.K. FA Davis Co., Philadelphia, PA, 1983.

Kinesiology and Applied Anatomy, 7th Ed. Rasch P.J. Williams & Wilkins, Baltimore, MD. 1989.

Anatomy of Movement. Calais-Germain B. Eastland Press, Inc. Seattle, WA. 1993.

Joint Structure and Function, A Comprehensive Analysis, 2nd Ed. Norkin C.C., Levangie P.K. FA Davis Co., Philadelphia, PA. 1992.

Neuromechanical Basis of Kinesiology, 2nd Ed. Enoka R.M. Human Kinetics Pub., Champaign, IL. 1994.

Manual of Structural Kinesiology, 12th Ed. Thompson C.W., Floyd R.T. Mosby-Year Book, Inc. Pub., St. Louis, MO. 1994.

Living Anatomy, 2nd Ed. Donnelly J.E. Human Kinetics Pub., Champaign, IL. 1990.

Applied Anatomy and Biomechanics in Sport. Bloomfield J., Ackland T.R., Elliott B.C. Human Kinetics Pub., Champaign, IL. 1994.

Coloring Guide to Regional Human Anatomy. Tweitmeyer A., McCracken T. Williams & Wilkins, Baltimore, MD.

Biomechanical Basis of Human Movement. Hamill J., Knutzen K.M. Williams & Wilkins, Baltimore, MD.

Kinetic Anatomy. Behnke, R.S. Human Kinetics Pub., Champaign, IL. 2001.

Personal Trainer Manual, The Resource for Fitness Professionals. Cotton R.T. (Ed.) American Council on Exercise, Pub. San Diego, CA. 2003.

Fitness: Theory & Practice, 3rd Ed. Published by AFAA (Sherman Oaks, CA). 2002.

ACSM Guidelines for Exercise Testing and Prescription, 6th Ed. Lippincott Williams & Wilkins, Baltimore, MD. 2000.

ACSM Resource Manual for Guidelines for Exercise Testing and Prescription. 3rd Ed. Williams & Wilkins, Baltimore, MD. 1998.

Health Fitness Instructor's Handbook, 4th Ed. Howley E.T., Franks B.D. Human Kinetics Pub., Champaign, IL. 2003.

Essentials of Strength Training and Conditioning, 3rd Ed. Baechle T.R. (Ed.) Human Kinetics Pub., Champaign, IL. 2003.

A Guide to Personal Fitness Training. Yoke MM. AFAA, Pub., Sherman Oaks, CA. 2001.

Athletic Injuries and Rehabilitation. Zachazewski J.E., Magee D.J., Quillen W.S. WB Saunders Co., Philadelphia, PA. 1996.

Biomechanics of Musculoskeletal Injury. Whiting W.C., Zernicke R.F. Human Kinetics Pub., Champaign, IL. 1998.

Designing Resistance Training Programs. Fleck S.J., Kraemer W.J. Human Kinetics Pub., Champaign, IL. 1987.

Weight Training Instruction: Steps to Success. Baechle T.R., Groves B.R. Human Kinetics Pub., Champaign, IL. 1994.

Strength Fitness, 3rd Ed. Westcott W. Wm. C. Brown Pub., Dubuque, IA. 1991.

Explosive Power and Strength. Chu D.A. Human Kinetics Pub., Champaign, IL. 1996.

Muscle Mechanics. Aaberg, E. Human Kinetics Pub., Champaign, IL. 1998.

Resistance Training Instruction. Aaberg, E. Human Kinetics Pub., Champaign, IL. 1999.

Back Stability. Norris C.M. Human Kinetics Pub., Champaign, IL. 2000.

Serious Strength Training. Bompa T.O., Cornacchia L.J. Human Kinetics Pub., Champaign, IL. 1998.

Jumping into Plyometrics. Chu D.A. Human Kinetics Pub., Champaign, IL. 1998.

Closed Kinetic Chain Exercise: A Comprehensive Guide to Multiple-Joint Exercises. Ellenbecker T.S., Davies G.J. Human Kinetics Pub., Champaign, IL. 2001.

Strength Ball Training. Goldenberg L., Twist P. Human Kinetics Pub., Champaign, IL. 2002.

Functional Training. Santana JC. JC Santana Pub., Boca Raton, FL. 2000.

Client Centered Exercise Prescription. Griffin J.D. Human Kinetics Pub., Champaign, IL. 1998.

Fitness Professionals' Guide to Musculoskeletal Anatomy and Human Movement. Golding, L.A., Golding S.M. Healthy Learning, Monterey, CA. 2003.

Mary Yoke, M.A. received her masters degree in exercise physiology from Adelphi University where she did her thesis research on the energy expenditure levels of specific group-fitness modalities. She also holds a bachelors and a masters degree in music. She holds 19 fitness certifications, including those from ACSM, AFAA, ACE, NASM, Stott Pilates, Physical Mind Institute, Yogafit, and Spinning. She is an adjunct professor at Adelphi University in New York, teaches group exercise and trains clients at a health club in Connecticut, travels nationally and internationally training fitness professionals, and presents wellness seminars to the general public. Professionally, she has worked in the areas of cardiac rehab, physical therapy, corporate fitness, and health promotion. She is a master trainer, specialist, and adjunct board member for AFAA, as well as a former member of ACSM's certification and credentialing committee. She is the author of *A Guide to Personal Fitness Training*.

Carol Kennedy, M.S. is certified by ACE and ACSM and is a faculty member in the Department of Kinesiology at Indiana University. She received her BS in leisure studies at the University of Illinois/Champaign/Urbana. She earned her MS in exercise science at Colorado State University where her thesis was based on research that she conducted in the area of water exercise. She has helped create and develop courses for the fitness specialist undergraduate degree program at IU. At IU, she teaches classes on group leadership, personal training, and general wellness. In her professional career, she has taught/created courses at three major universities within the United States and has produced several instructional videos on water exercise and functional exercise progression. She has written a well-received book on group leadership. She is a former member of the ACSM certification and credentialing committee and has presented both nationally and internationally on various fitness/wellness topics.

About the Authors